PENGUIN BOOKS

YOGA ALSO FOR THE GODLESS

Born Mumtaz Ali in Thiruvananthapuram, Kerala, Sri M is a spiritual teacher, author, social reformer, educationist and global speaker. His memoir, *Apprenticed to a Himalayan Master: A Yogi's Autobiography*, published in 2011, became an instant bestseller; the sequel, *The Journey Continues*, was published in 2017.

He is the author of various other books on philosophy, yoga and Indian mysticism. Sri M established The Satsang Foundation twenty years ago and his mission has resulted in several initiatives in areas of education, community health, environment and the oneness of humanity.

Among the many awards and honours he has received, Sri M was conferred the Padma Bhushan by the Government of India in January 2020 for distinguished service of high order in spirituality.

YOGA
ALSO FOR THE GODLESS

SRI M

PENGUIN BOOKS
An imprint of Penguin Random House

PENGUIN BOOKS

USA | Canada | UK | Ireland | Australia
New Zealand | India | South Africa | China

Penguin Books is part of the Penguin Random House group of companies
whose addresses can be found at global.penguinrandomhouse.com

Published by Penguin Random House India Pvt. Ltd
4th Floor, Capital Tower 1, MG Road,
Gurugram 122 002, Haryana, India

Penguin
Random House
India

First published by Westland Publications Private Limited in 2020
This edition published in Penguin Books by Penguin Random House India in 2022

10 9 8 7 6 5 4 3 2 1

The views and opinions expressed in this book are the author's own and the
facts are as reported by him which have been verified to the extent possible,
and the publishers are not in any way liable for the same.

ISBN 9780143458593

Typeset by Jojy Philip, New Delhi - 110015

www.penguin.co.in

CONTENTS

WHY THIS BOOK?

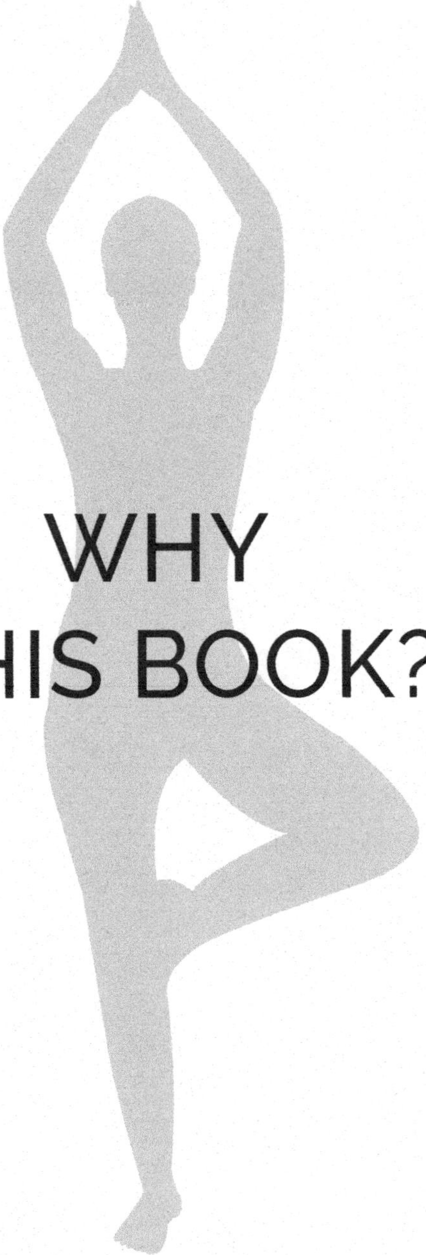

There is no knowledge equal to Sankhya and no power equal to yoga.

—Mahabharata

Some years ago, I met a smart young lady who said to me, 'M, I believe you are a yogi. I think you might be able to shed light on a question on yoga. I was very keen on practising yoga after I heard about its health benefits. The fact that many celebrities practise yoga to keep in shape also influenced me.

'I approached a yoga teacher. He started teaching me Sanskrit shlokas in praise of God and insisted that I chant them. I tried convincing him that I was an atheist. I was born a Hindu but do not think it necessary to believe in God. He strongly felt that without invoking Lord Ganesha, I could not begin my yoga practice and insisted that the aim of yoga was God-realisation.

'I told him that there is no God and, therefore, learning yoga for me was not to reach something that, according to me, did not exist. He was adamant and asked me to find another instructor'.

'What do you think?'

*

This yoga teacher, the girl referred to, is not an exception. Thousands of people labour under the mistaken notion that yoga is a theistic philosophy and is not for atheists and agnostics. Some yoga teachers admit that mere postures can provide health benefits, but the higher aspects such as the expansion of consciousness and the attainment of *Kaivalya*, freeing the consciousness from the limitations of conditioned thinking and awakening to its infinite potential, is not realisable by the godless.

This book is meant precisely to change such misunderstood notions about yoga, while serving as a practical guide to practise yoga to perfection, without the 'God crutch'. You will understand that ancient yoga philosophy has almost no interest in the concept of a creator or an all-powerful God, who controls you and throws you into heaven or hell according to his whims and fancies.

Even the great Patanjali, considered the foremost and earliest exponent of systematic yoga, in his masterpiece, *The Yoga Sutras*, uses *Ishwara* (God) only twice in the entire text and only as a useful adjunct to the main practices. Whether Patanjali's Ishwara denotes an omnipotent 'thundering God' or the tranquil *Purusha* of *Sankhya* philosophy is an age-old question that needs a healthy debate. We will look into these and other points of view because to practise yoga well, an understanding of its philosophical roots is important.

Lastly, this book is an attempt to save the purity of yoga from being adulterated by religious cults and politico-religious outfits keen to exploit the masses and use them to their advantage.

AN INTRODUCTION TO YOGA

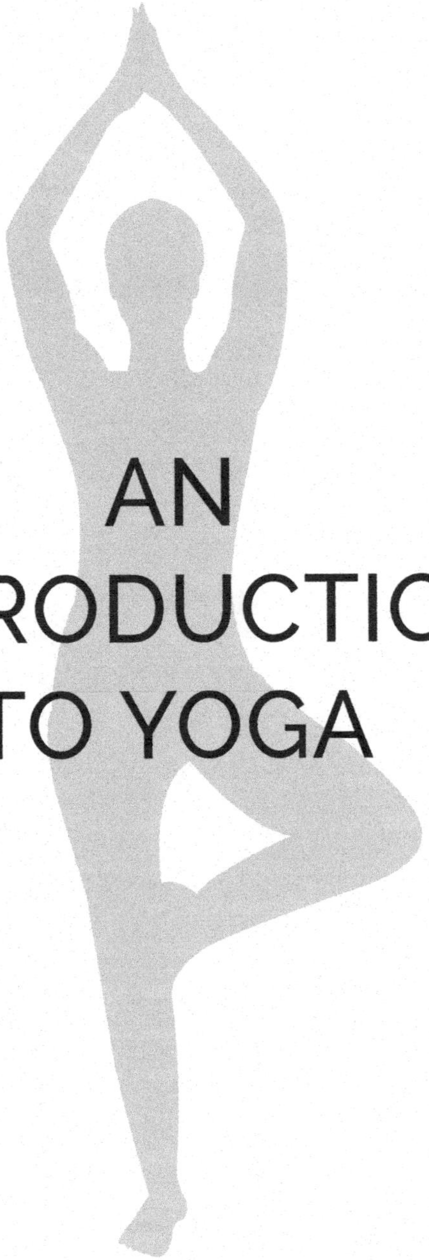

Yoga is an ancient science included in the six *darshanas*[1] of traditional Indian philosophy. While the theoretical concepts are mostly derived from Sankhya, there are a few differences, particularly regarding the concept of Ishwara. One important difference is that while Sankhya offers a purely philosophical framework, yoga while using Sankhya terminology goes into the practical steps of achieving the goal, which Sankhya envisages only theoretically. The relationship between Sankhya and yoga can be compared to the relationship between science and technology. Scientific theories are abstract, while technology actualises such theories into tangible findings and useful results.

However, technology sometimes exploits the findings for nefarious and destructive purposes. It is to offset this danger that the practice of moral principles is harmonised with that of yoga at the very beginning. The most important moral principle is *ahimsa*, or non-injury to living beings, including humans. The yogi acquires tremendous energy and almost unlimited knowledge as the practice frees the brain of burdens, disturbances and conflicts, resulting in tranquillity and one-pointedness. By adhering to moral principles, the yogi's energy and knowledge are not misdirected for selfish purposes.

---

[1] Coming face to face with reality would be a fair translation of the Sanskrit word *darshana*.

Banishing petty ego, is, therefore, a prime moral constituent of the yogic system and practice.

Sankhya, a dualistic philosophy, postulates Purusha, which is pure consciousness, and *Prakriti,* which is primordial matter that transforms into the material world. Prakriti defined as *Prakarotiti Prakriti,* that which divides, is responsible for the diversity of the universe. In the human organism, as in the universe, Purusha is the consciousness and Prakriti, the material part, including the body and thoughts originating from the brain. Yoga admits of a special Purusha called Ishwara who guides evolution and which the tranquil and purified mind of the yogi soon identifies with his own Purusha component.

The definition of yoga in *The Yoga Sutras of Patanjali,* the ancient authority on yoga, is *yogas chitta vritti nirodha.* Translated, this means the art of clearing the mind of all distractions and conflicts. Enlightenment or Kaivalya, the culmination of yogic practices, occurs when the mind frees itself from the conditioning influence of Prakriti and enjoys its original, infinite freedom and bliss resting in Purusha alone. Kaivalya could be defined as aloneness in the midst of the multiplicity of daily existence, the direct result of the perfect stillness of the mind that the yogi acquires. To put it differently, it means the mind is set free from limitations and experiences vastness and all-pervasiveness. The yogi looks upon sorrow and disappointment with equanimity, and neither touches him. Such a yogi may retire or work for the welfare of humanity, without any hint of self-centredness. This is the goal of yoga.

God, as we usually conceive him, has no role to play in this transformation. Significantly, even in *The Yoga Sutras of Patanjali*, the word Ishwara only appears in a couple of shlokas. As the philosophical foundations are mostly derived from Sankhya, the meaning of the term Ishwara becomes ambiguous. Although Sankhya refers to a special Purusha, that Purusha is understood as being no different from the Purusha component of the individual, once Prakriti has been shed. This concept has given birth to the theory that an advanced yogi who has ascended to the aloneness of Kaivalya is himself Ishwara, the Lord. The corollary to this is that if one's teacher or instructor—I am overriding the word Guru deliberately, since it is so loaded—has reached Kaivalya, he may be the one to be addressed as Ishwara, from whom help may be sought.

I must add that in the 'Samadhi Pada', a chapter in *The Yoga Sutras*, Patanjali states that one of the ways of attaining *samadhi*—the Superconscious state that leads to Kaivalya, the ultimate goal—is by meditation on the concept of Ishwara. *Ishwara pranidhanatva* is the actual sutra in Sanskrit. Aside from what Ishwara could mean, from what we have already discussed about the term, the *va* at the end of the sutra needs further understanding. It also means one of the many techniques that is not given special importance. One of the many ways is 'contemplation on the Ishwara'—this would be quite an accurate description.

Although the Buddhists of the Yogachara school are atheists, they also visualise and invoke deities in their meditation techniques. This shows that these are mostly methods adopted to quieten the mind ultimately and that the deities, in this case, are given the stature of an almighty supreme creator and destroyer God. Significantly, a sutra in the Patanjali text that is placed close to the previous one is *oushadhanam*, literally meaning 'taking chemical substances'. If oushadhanam is also one of the ways for altering states of consciousness, leading to samadhi, this speaks for itself.

To reach this goal of Kaivalya, yoga teaches a step-by-step approach. *The Yoga Sutras*, which are referred to as a treatise of Kriya Yoga, including by the author himself, is also known as Ashtanga Yoga, the yoga of the eight limbs. It describes *yama* and *niyama*, the rules and regulations to be followed, which begin with ahimsa—non-injury to living beings and, in general, advocate moderation in diet and in all walks of life, and simple living. It goes on to *asanas* (postures), *pranayama* (regulation of breath), *pratyahara* (developing the capacity to withdraw the sense organs at will), *dharana* (one-pointed attention), *dhyana* (meditation) and finally, samadhi (the state in which the mind is set free of all conditioning and realises its full potential).

The single-most important precept of the *Śramaṇa*, who later were also referred to as *jinas*, is *ahimsa paramo dharma*. Their greatest virtue is that of non-injury to other living beings. This is not a moral precept or a part of a divine revelation, given that they are confirmed atheists. But this is to be practised in daily life so as to purify the mind and lead it to nirvana.

Going back to the eight steps, asanas or body postures, though they often look like gymnastic exercises, are not merely for physical well-being, but are also designed to activate and modulate the functioning of the endocrine system. The asanas play a major role in regulating and altering moods, leading to the ability to avoid sudden mood swings and achieving balance and tranquillity. *Pranayama* or the regulation of breath also plays a major role in keeping the body supplied with the right quantity of oxygen, while at the same time, calming down the mind and turning it inward to a tranquil, meditative state.

*

Having come so far, the reader would have, perhaps, found the answer to the question—can yoga be practised by an atheist or agnostic? Anyone who has taken up the practice of yoga is sure to benefit in many ways, especially in finding tranquillity and peace in this tumultuous world and in being able to harness tremendous energy.

To sum up, excellence in yoga, the science of expansion of consciousness and achieving freedom from limitation, has nothing to do with one's personal beliefs, religious or otherwise. It depends entirely on the step-by-step practice of the methods described in the yoga texts and guidance of a proper and authentic expert. To take up the practice of yoga based on having read up an obscure text, without the guidance of an expert, is fraught with danger, and the physical and psychological consequences can be serious. If, on the other hand, one is patient and goes at it carefully, taking up only those practices that suit one's physical and mental capacity, a great new world, vast and almost unlimited, opens up before the yogi, who turns into one of the finest specimens of homo sapiens, with an inexhaustible fund of energy and a mind at peace. An authentic yoga teacher, open to dialogue and not intent on forming a cult, would be ideal in helping customise one's yoga practice.

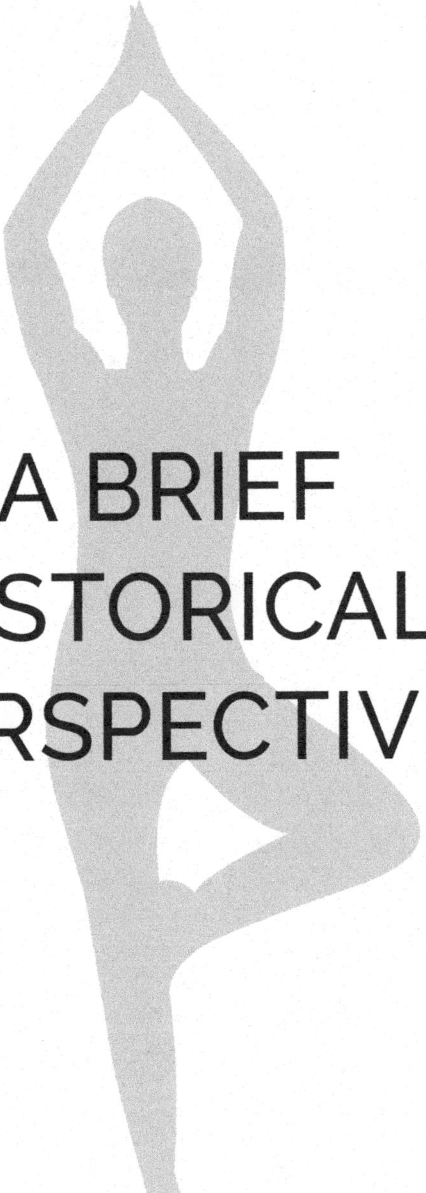

A BRIEF HISTORICAL PERSPECTIVE

Not giving too much importance to a creator God and the tilt towards atheism is not a later-day invention, but is already evident in the Sankhya, the works of the Shravanas and the Buddhists and, to a great extent, in *The Yoga Sutras*, itself. Much before the epics made their appearance and a belief in the incarnations of God became almost a creed in the Hindu systems of thought, the great Vedic hymns and the Upanishads later, celebrated free thought and a non-conformist rational attitude.

The earliest example from the Nasadiya Sukta of the *Rig Veda*, the first of the four Vedas considered *shruti* or the original fountainhead of wisdom, as the Hymn of Creation. Parts of it read like a description of the origin of the cosmos in scientific works. The foremost point is the healthy spirit of scepticism throughout. Here is an excellent translation of the *Hymn of Creation* (Book 10: CXXIX), *Rig Veda* by Ralph T.H. Griffith. Having read the original in Sanskrit, I can vouch for its accuracy.

The Hymn of Creation

1. THEN was not non-existent nor existent: there was no realm of air, no sky beyond it.
   What covered in, and where? And what gave shelter? Was water there, unfathomed depth of water?

2. Death was not then, nor was there aught immortal: no sign

was there, the day's and night's divider. That One Thing, breathless, breathed by its own nature: apart from it was nothing whatsoever.

3. Darkness there was: at first concealed in darkness this All was indiscriminate chaos.

   All that existed then was void and formless: by the great power of warmth was born that unit.

4. Thereafter rose desire at the beginning. Desire, the primal seed and germ of spirit.

   Sages who searched with their heart's thought discovered the existent's kinship in the non-existent.

5. Transversely was their severing line extended: what was above it then, and what below it?

   There were begetters, there were mighty forces, free action here and energy up yonder.

6. Who verily knows and who can here declare it, whence it was born and whence comes this creation? The Gods are later than this world's production. Who knows then whence it first came into being?

7. He, the first origin of this creation, whether he formed it all or did not form it.

   Whose eye controls this world in highest heaven, he verily knows it, or perhaps he knows not.

To be specifically noted are the number of question marks and the fourth, sixth and seventh shlokas, which can be related to the practice of yoga.

SHANTI MANTRA

Now let's take a look at some of the shanti mantras that occur in the Upanishads, the core and essence of the Vedas. They are mostly assertions, affirmations and wishes to ascend spiritually and derive physical and mental strength to achieve the goals, rather than through prayers to an almighty creator. Many of them end with the sincere wish for peace—shanti—and the wish to improve the world and the beings that live in it.

Asatomā sadgamaya
From the unreal may I ascend to the real,

Tamaso mā jyotirgamaya
From darkness, may I ascend to light,

Mṛtyor mā amṛtaṃ gamaya
From death may I ascend to deathlessness,

Oṁ[2] śhānti śhānti śhāntiḥ
Om! Peace, peace, peace.

*

Om sarve bhavantu sukhinah
May all be happy,

---

[2] In Chapter 5, the sound of Om is discussed in detail.

Sarve santu nirāmayāḥ
May all be free from illness,

Sarve bhadrāṇi paśyantu
May all see what is auspicious,

Mā kashcid duḥkha bhāgbhavet
May there be no suffering,

Oṁ shānti shānti, śhāntiḥ
Om! Peace, peace, peace.

⁎

Oṁ Sahanā vavatu
May we both be protected (the teacher and the taught),

Saha nau bhunaktu
May we both obtain nourishment,

Saha vīryam karavāvahai
May we work together with vigour and vitality,

Tejasvi nāvadhītamastu
May we be lit with the light of wisdom,

Mā vidviṣāvahai
May we not quarrel and argue with each other,

Oṁ shānti shānti, śhāntiḥ
Om! Peace, peace, peace.

*

Ōm pūrṇam adaḥ pūrṇam idam
Om that is complete, this is complete,

Pūrṇāt pūrṇamudacyate
From completeness has come completeness,

Pūrṇasya pūrṇamādāya
When this completeness is taken from that completeness,

Pūrṇamevā vaśiṣyate
Completeness only remains,

Oṁ shānti shānti, śhāntiḥ
Om! Peace, peace, peace.

*

In the above mantra, there is no reference to a creator God. It is a statement of completeness or fullness of the truth or ultimate reality. Sankhya and yoga would call it the fullness of Purusha, our true being when free from the conditioning of Prakriti, the world of matter. Vedantists would prefer the word *Brahman*, all that remains after the negation of all tangible objects.

The goal of yoga is to find that fullness of the eternally free Purusha, rarely called Ishwara in one's own Self, freed of all conditioning caused by Prakriti.

YOGA IN ANCIENT TEACHINGS

Let's move to the earliest references to yoga in the ancient teachings. The first reference to yoga in the Upanishads, the Brahmanical texts, occurs in the *Katha Upanishad.*

Katha Upanishad: Restraint of the senses—when the five senses (instruments of knowledge) and the mind remain still, not active, it is known as the highest state. Yoga is considered as the restraint of the senses. Then one is undistracted, for yoga is the rising and the passing away.

Then the Bhagavad Gita:

Tranquillity and skilled action:

- Perform actions established in yoga. Give up attachment, Arjuna. Treat success and failure as equal. Yoga is equanimity.
- Yoga is to be skilled in action.
- Yoga is separation from contact with suffering.
- The yogi is superior to the ascetics, superior to those who have the knowledge, even to the ritualists. Be a yogi, Arjuna.

The Mahabharata says:

There is no power equal to yoga. No knowledge equal to Sankhya.

Then there are a number of Yogachara texts of the Buddhists. The *Yogācārabhūmi-Śāstra* is one among many texts that deal with yoga. There is also a body of *Sramana* literature linked to the ancient Jaina school of thought that elaborates on yogic practices. The Yogachara school, it should be noted, pre-dates Patanjali's *Yoga Sutras*. The classic definition of yoga in *The Yoga Sutras* is:

'Yoga is the stopping of the distractions of the mind.' It could also be translated as the suppression of the activities of the mind. There are several other texts on yoga, most of them written after Patanjali's *Yoga Sutras*. We do not need to go into them at the moment and will bring them in when appropriate, as we proceed.

Given below are some of the titles:

(i) *Vaiśeṣika Sutra*
(ii) *Malinivijayottara Tantra*
(iii) *Shiva Purana*
(iv) *Vyasa's commentary on the Yoga Sutras of Patanjali*
(v) *Vasistha Samhita*
(vi) *Yogasastra of Hemachandra*
(vii) *Yoga Bija*
(viii) *Hamsavilasa of Sri Hamsamithu*
(ix) *Gheranda Samhita*
(x) *Goraksha Shataka*
(xi) *Yoga Pradipika*
(xii) *Yoga Yajnavalkya*

There is a fair amount of controversy surrounding the dates of these texts; however, it is not relevant to the discussion. Before ending this chapter, here is a quotation from the Bhagavad Gita, which endorses my view that the *Yoga Darshana* is by and large, not very different from the *Sankhya Darshana*, though yoga lays more stress on practice.

'The foolish declare that Sankhya and yoga are separate. Not the wise. He who performs even one of them correctly obtains the fruit of both. The state attained by the Sankhyas is also attained by the yogis. Sankhya and yoga are one. Who knows this truly knows'—The Bhagavad Gita.

Sankhya is not an atheistic philosophy.

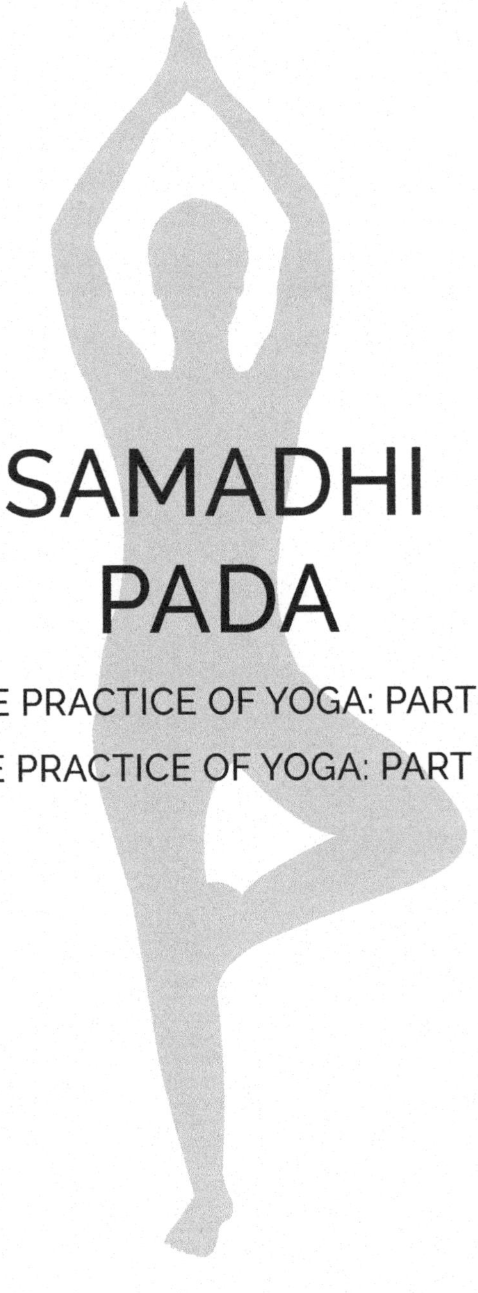

SAMADHI PADA

THE PRACTICE OF YOGA: PART I

THE PRACTICE OF YOGA: PART II

THE PRACTICE OF YOGA

PART I

We have discussed the question of whether the concept of a creator God—Ishwara—is an intrinsic part of the yoga of Patanjali and found that it is not so. We can now proceed to the theory, and above all, the practice of yoga. Please note that even in Sankhya and in the Buddhist and Jain teachings, the idea of a creator God plays no role.

Patanjali begins with the rather terse sutra, *Atha Yoga Anushasanam*. Now begins the practise of Yoga.

Let's start with:

1. Samadhi Pada: The study of the Superconscious state.
2. Sadhana Pada: The actual practice.
3. Vibhuti Pada: The extraordinary attainments achieved by the practice.
4. Kaivalya Pada: The ultimate freedom realised by the practitioner on attaining the highest goal—the power of extraordinary awareness and freedom from conditioning.

The choice of belief in Ishwara is entirely the initiate's prerogative. Let me reiterate that belief in Ishwara is not a prerequisite for success in Yoga, even to reach the highest level of Kaivalya.

In addition to *The Yoga Sutras*, we will refer to other post-Patanjali texts like the *Shiva Samhita* and *Yoga Yagnavalkya*, among others, whenever required to supplement our learning. The Upanishads, including the earliest principal Upanishads and the later *Yoga Upanishads*, will also form a part of our reference material.

SAMADHI PADA

Let's take up the classic sutra of Patanjali, which is the second one after 'Now, the instruction in yoga': *yogas chitta vritti nirodha*, which literally translated would mean, 'Yoga is the restraint of the modifications of the *chitta*.' Different translators have used 'fluctuations', 'distortions,' and so on, to explain it. But it is necessary to understand the word chitta before comprehending the word *nirodha*, mostly translated as restrain.

Many translations have used the word 'mind-stuff'. But my submission is that if Patanjali meant mind-stuff, the appropriate equivalent word should have been *mano vritti*. I would prefer to use the more factual word, brain, for chitta. *Vritti* means activity, modifications, fluctuations, among other words.

The brain is not static. It is intensely dynamic at its core. But regular brain activity, marked by attractions and repulsions linked to the objective sensory world, keeps the brain so distracted that it has no time to reach in to its core, because of the fluctuations that it feels.

When these distractions and fluctuations disappear, the components of the incessant movement of thought are silenced and eradicated. The brain no longer dissipates energy and settles into a silent, deep and tranquil state, which is its real core, says Patanjali. In this state, the yogi is filled with tremendous energy, experiencing bliss and fullness.

The quiet and tranquil brain is empowered with the highest intelligence and becomes capable of rising to the fullness of Superconsciousness.

As soon as the external and internal activities of the brain are curbed, collective wisdom is realised. Free of the burden of useless information, the brain turns inwards and realises its full potential. As the brain is now clear of all the past debris, it becomes creative and subtle.

According to yoga, the core of our consciousness has all the knowledge and wisdom 'a priori' within itself. Wisdom is not acquired from outside but is revealed from within when various conditionings are removed. The key to unlocking this vast, almost omniscient potential is yoga.

The third shloka aptly describes a yogi's state as: *tada drastah sva rupe vasthanam.* 'Then there is the abiding in the Seer's own original form.' To put it simply, when fluctuations and distractions cease with yoga practice, one realises that one is the Seer, pure and blissful—not the 'seen', which is only part of life's drama.

The yogi realises that he doesn't possess consciousness but is consciousness itself. She/he is no longer confined to the brain's limited thought processes, which have, indeed, been successfully transcended. The yogi is now divine and needs no divinity or deity as a crutch.

Before we move on to Part II of Chapter 4, here is an important clarification:

The etymological Sanskrit root of the word *yoga* is *yuj-a* i.e., concentration and *yuj-i* is conjunction. In various books, yoga is interpreted as being synonymous with the English word 'yoke'. This interpretation is incorrect. In fact, yoga's goal is to get rid of all yokes so that the brain can return to its core—pure consciousness.

Another mistaken notion is that yoga is the joining of the Individual Self (*jivatma)* and the Universal Self (*paramatma)*. Nowhere does Sankhya or yoga refer to jivatma and paramatma or the uniting of the two.

This simplistic definition is a result of the confusion of linking the yoga system with other philosophies and religious cults, which have borrowed extensively from yoga.

There is no mystic union of man and God in yoga. Rather, man is exhorted to know himself by silencing the brain and reaching into the core of consciousness, where he recognises himself as Purusha, the blissful ever-free Seer of all that is visible and invisible.

The false belief in a separate ego, different from others, is put to rest, and one abides as the one universal Purusha, severed from pain—as the Gita states. The root of all conflict that stems from the narrow individual ego-sense is banished forever. The yogi is now free.

THE PRACTICE OF YOGA
PART II

Sutra 4

vṛtti sārūpyam itaratra

At other times (when not tranquil and therefore not established in its original state of the Seer) the brain takes the form of fluctuations, conflict and agitation.

Sutra 5

vṛttayaḥ pañcatayyaḥ kliṣṭākliṣṭāḥ

There are five-fold fluctuations; those that are painful and tormenting and those that are pleasurable, but all the same, fluctuations.

Patanjali then goes on to enumerate the five types of fluctuations.

1. Valid knowledge (*pramana*)
2. Misconceptions or illusions (*viparyaya*)
3. Delusion consisting of mere words (*vikalpa*)
4. Sleep (*nidra*)
5. Memory (*smriti*)

To sum up, outward as well as inward activities keep the brain engaged and constantly in motion. Valid knowledge means knowledge arrived at by processing the data gathered by the sense organs of sight, hearing, taste, smell and touch.

Unfortunately, the instruments of perception have a limited range and many-a-time provide incorrect data as in the case of optical illusions. The so-called valid knowledge arrived at, based on these inputs, is not reliable; but the brain tends to accept it at face value, and the consequent pleasure or pain causes terrible fluctuations, which prevent the brain from settling down.

Those misconceptions, which are based again on the limited capacity of the instruments of perception wherein an illusion is seen as a reality or the reality is seen as an illusion, is the second category, *viparyaya*. A rope in the dark, mistaken as a snake with the consequent reaction of panic, is a good example of the second category used by the Buddhists as well as by Vedantins.

Verbal delusion is the one caused by using words to exaggerate feelings. The literature of romantic and devotional poetry, where hyperbolic expressions are used to heighten emotion, is a classic example of verbal delusion. Even commercial cinema falls in this category. Seeing the exaggeration deliberately created by dialogues, songs, music and special effects, the viewer tends to imitate the drama in real life and often lives in a world of delusion.

Sleep is a category of fluctuations, which forms part of lethargy. While sleep is needed to rejuvenate one daily, the yogi transcends the need for too much sleep. Free of the *tamo guna*, his brain settles down into conscious tranquillity, which is in contrast to the rest, felt due to the absence of conscious awareness in sleep.

Memory, too, is a cause of fluctuations. There is a constant struggle to avoid bitter memories and hold on to pleasant ones, forgetting that both are memories, which are mere recordings in the brain and not the reality that is here and now.

The yogi treats pleasant and unpleasant memories as just memories and transcends the need to either hold on to one or avoid the other. In a yogic state, fluctuations caused by memory cease.

*

Many of the sutras up to the eleventh one are explanations and elaborations of the different kinds of fluctuations.

Sutra 12

abhyāsa-vairāgya-ābhyāṁ tan-nirodhaḥ

Through practise and dispassion arises restraint.

Dispassion, simply put, means not being at the mercy of passions. A dispassionate person is one who has learnt to restrain himself from actions, which in the long run, cause pain, though they may seem pleasurable at first.

When one is firmly situated in a dispassionate space, the brain instead of moving towards becoming, learns to be. When this is uninterrupted, the real identity called the Purusha comes to the fore.

Yoga practitioners are categorised as mild, medium and intense.

Sutra 20

śraddhā-vīrya-smṛti samādhi-prajñā-pūrvaka itareṣām

Those who have faith in the practice, energy and mindfulness, move towards the Superconscious state called samadhi that culminates in wisdom.

Sutra 23

īśvara-praṇidhānād-vā

This can happen (note the syllable *va*, which means also) also by dedication to Ishwara.

Sutra 24

kleśa karma vipākāśayaiḥ-aparāmṛṣṭaḥ puruṣa-viśeṣa īśvaraḥ

It is a distinct Purusha, untouched by afflictions, actions, fruitions or their residue.

Sutra 25

tatra niratiśayaṁ sarvajña-bījam

There the seed of Omniscience is unsurpassed.

As we have discussed at length the concept of Ishwara according to Patanjali in the first chapter itself, there is no need to go into elaborate details. But a few points are to be noted.

1. That dedication to Ishwara is only considered one of the ways or psychological procedures to attain samadhi. Once more, note the word *va*.

2. To distinguish the Ishwara mentioned here from a creator and protector God akin to the Semitic God or the Gods of the several Puranas, Patanjali hastens to add that Ishwara means a distinct Purusha untouched by afflictions, actions, fruitions or their residue, but blessed with the seed of unsurpassed Omniscience.

   This makes the concept of Ishwara the same as that of the primordial Purusha of Sankhya, an atheistic philosophy, as already mentioned. The yogi ultimately realises that in essence, he is indeed that Purusha or Ishwara.

3. Therefore, it could also mean a yogi who has touched the highest samadhi and attained the exalted state of Ishwara.

4. Although Patanjali emphasises relying only on one's own efforts, the suggestion is that a perfected yogi as well as devotion or surrendering to the Supreme Purusha would help.

Sutra 26

sa eṣa pūrveṣām api-guruḥ kālena-anavacchedāt

Due to it being unlimited by time, it is the teacher of the ones who came before.

Which means that this timeless Ishwara, the Purusha has been considered a teacher by the yogis of yore.

Sutra 27

tasya vācakaḥ praṇavaḥ

The manifest expansion of this sublime Ishwara is the *Pranava* (*Om*).

Sutra 28

tad japas tad-artha-bhāvanam

Therefore, repetition of it and the realisation of its purpose should be made.

Sutra 29

tataḥ pratyak-cetana-adhigamo-`py-antarāya-abhavaś-ca

This inward consciousness is attained, and obstacles do not arise.

Since the meaning of the word *Om* and the procedure involved in the repetition of it and the results need a great deal of elaboration, this is dealt with in the next chapter.

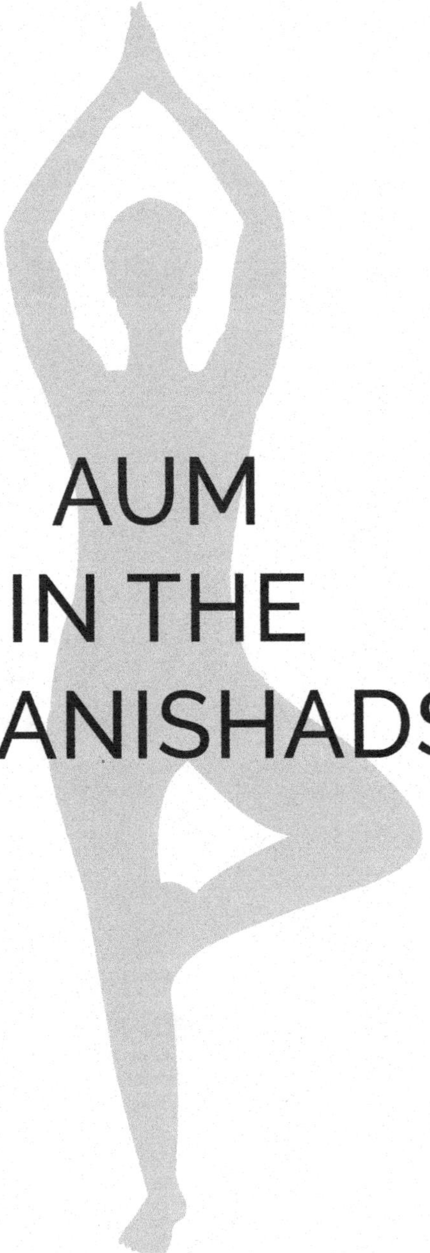

AUM IN THE UPANISHADS

In Sutras 27, 28 and 29, mentioned at the end of Chapter 4, Part II, which deals with *Om* and also mentions the effect of chanting it, Patanjali draws from sources as ancient as the Upanishads.

Among the Principal Upanishads that deal with *Pranava* or Om, the *Katha Upanishad*, the *Mundaka* and the *Mandukya* stand out distinctly. In fact, the *Mandukya* is an exposition of the Principle of Om, which is spelt AUM. It belongs to the *Atharva Veda.*

The *Mandukya Upanishad* has earned the distinction of being commented upon by Gaudapada, Shankara's teacher. Equally significantly, it is considered as perhaps the first systematic exposition of the non-dual system called *Advaita Vedanta.* The *karika* of Gaudapada is so close to the *Shunya Vada* of the aesthetic Buddhists that some surmise that Gaudapada was a Buddhist.

The prolific Shankara has commented on both the Upanishad and the karika of Gaudapada. Interestingly, even Shankara was labelled a *prachanna Boudhika* (Buddhist in disguise) by one section of the orthodoxy of the ancient city of Varanasi.

As the *Mandukya Upanishad* consists of just 12 shlokas, it is inarguably the shortest of the Upanishads. Significantly, there is no mention of Ishwara in it. Importantly, it addresses the different states of consciousness common to all human beings, represented by the syllables A, U and M of the sacred *Aum.*

Shloka 1

aum ity etad akṣaram idam sarvam,
tasyopavyākhyānam bhūtam bhavad
bhaviṣyad iti sarvam auṁkāra eva yac
cānyat trikālātītaṁ tad apy auṁkāra eva

Aum, this syllable is all this. The explanation is as follows: All that is the past, the present and the future, all this is the syllable Aum. And that which is beyond the threefold time, that too is only the syllable Aum.

The Aum which is the syllable of Brahman, the ultimate reality, stands for the manifested world, the past, present and future, and also the unmanifested Absolute.

Shloka 2

sarvaṁ hy etad brahma, ayam ātmā
brahma so'yam ātmā chatuṣ-pāt

All this is, verily Brahman. My inner Self is Brahman. This Self appears to have four quarters.

One needs to only replace the word Brahman with Purusha to see that when Patanjali talks of the Purusha being the true essence of the Self, free from all conditionings and distractions of the chitta that obscure it, the difference is only in terminology.

Shloka 3

jāgarita sthāno bahiṣ-prajñaḥ saptāṅga
ekonaviṁśati-mukha sthūla-bhug
vaiśvānaraḥ prathamaḥ pādah

> The first quarter is *vaishvanara*, whose sphere is the waking state, who cognises external objects, who has seven limbs and nineteen mouths and enjoys the gross, material objects.

The nineteen mouths are the five sense organs (sight, hearing, touch, taste and smell), the five organs of action (speech, the use of limbs, movement, generation, excretion), the five vital breaths—*pranas, manas* (the mind), *buddhi* (the intellect), *ahamkara* (the sense of recognising oneself) and chitta, the entire sphere of thought that encompasses everything.

The waking state, therefore, represented by **A** (Aum), is the normal condition experienced by all humans.

Shloka 4

> *svapna-sthāno'ntaḥ-prajñaḥ saptāṅga*
> *ekonavimśati-mukhaḥ*
> *pravivikta-bhuk taijaso dvītiyaḥ pādah*

> The second quarter is *taijasa*, represented by **U** (Aum), whose sphere of activity is the dream state, which cognises internal objects and enjoys the subtle objects.

This is also common to all living beings, the dream state where one experiences with closed eyes, a world of imagination that originates from the sub-conscious and yet is so real that while dreaming, no one believes it is a dream. It is only when one wakes up that one says, 'O! What a dream.' Some sages declare that in the waking state, when one is not in deep sleep, life appears to be a living long-drawn dream. A person whose mind is still limited will not accept this. But when the mind expands, all distractions and conditions are removed and one experiences Absolute consciousness at the core of one's being, it may be seen as such.

The sage wakes up to reality and says, 'O! What a dream,' delightful or terrible as the case may be.

Shloka 5

eṣa sarveśvaraḥ eṣa sarvajñaḥ, eṣo'ntāryami, eṣa yoniḥ sarvasya prabhavāpyayau hi bhūtānām

Where one, being fast asleep, does not desire any desire whatsoever and does not see any dream, that is deep sleep. The third quarter is *pragna*, whose sphere is the state of deep sleep, who has become One, verily a mass of cognition, who is full of bliss, who enjoys bliss, whose face is thought.

So, in the state of deep sleep, where the diversity of cognition of outside objects and inside dreams have ceased and consciousness reverts to its unity, the Self, then is in a state of bliss, experiencing bliss not through indulgence, which depends on sense objects, but absorbed in its own intrinsic blissfulness, alone and independent.

Shloka 6

āntaḥ-prajñam, na bahiṣ prajñam, nobhayataḥ-prajñam
na prajnañā-ghanam, na prajñam, nāprajñam;
adṛṣtam, avyavahārayam, agrāhyam, alakṣaṇam,
acintyam, avyapadeśyam, ekātma-pratyaya-

> *sāram, prapañcopaśamam, śāntam, śivam, advaitam, caturtham manyante, sa ātmā, sa vijñeyaḥ*
>
> This is the Lord of all, this is the Knower of all, this is the inner controller; this is the source of all; this is the beginning and end of all beings.

Gaudapada in his karika says, '*Eka eva tridha smrtha*'. It is the one alone who is known in the three states.

Therefore, now the questions arise:

1. So if the Self is in the blissful state of deep sleep, in that state are we not aware of bliss, as we are in a state of unconsciousness?
2. And, is this the end? In which case, which is the fourth quarter? **A, U** and **M** seem to have been explained. Is there something more?

Before attempting to answer these questions, we should move to the next shloka.

Shloka 7

> *so'yam ātmādhyakṣaram*
> *auṁkaro'dhimātram pādā mātrā*
> *mātrāś ca pādā akāra ukāra makāra iti*
>
> *Turiya* is not that which cognises the internal objects nor the external objects, nor a mass of cognition yet non-cognitive. It is unseen, incapable of being spoken of, unpalpable, without any distinctive marks, unthinkable, unnamable, the essence of the knowledge of the one

> Self, that into which the word is resolved, the peaceful, benign, non-dual, such they think, is the fourth quarter. That is the Self: That is to be known.

No wonder Buddha called it *shunya*, zero, no-thing and Gaudapada, the great commentator was believed to have been a Buddhist.

Now to return to the questions:

1. One seems to be unaware of the bliss of the Self in a deep sleep, but surely there must have been someone who was aware of this bliss when one wakes up from a deep sleep, for there is always a remembrance of the blissfulness. The usual expression when we wake up from a deep, dreamless sleep is, 'O! What a blissful sleep.' The bliss lingers on, and one is likely to turn around and go back to sleep in an attempt to recapture the bliss, even when the wake-up alarm has rung many times.

So *sushupti* or deep sleep, the state in which one revels in the bliss of the Self, even if only temporarily, and because of which, one is rejuvenated and ready for the day, is nature's indicator of the presence of the Supreme Self. This Self nudges one on to figure out if one can experience the blissful Self while being fully conscious, at a time when everything else conforms to the deep sleep state.

If, and the yogis say it is possible, such a state can be realised, that will be the supremely blissful and Superconscious state called turiya, the last quarter of the Pranava, which the Yoga Darshana calls Kaivalya.

2. While it is true that when Aum is written as **A, U** and **M** in English, it has only three parts but written in Devanagari, this is how it looks—ॐ. Now, the last sound 'M' doesn't end abruptly, but continues in a sort of hum, like the sound of a bell or a gong that continues for some time and then fades away into a frequency that can no longer be detected by our instrument of hearing, the ear. The term used to describe this is *ardhamatra*.

(We will deal with the practical aspects of repeating Aum, as mentioned in Sutra 28 of the Samadhi Pada of Patanjali that was referred to earlier, at the end of the chapter).

It is this almost imperceptible part of ॐ that is the fourth quarter and represents turiya, that cannot be grasped by the physical senses, but which is realised when the mind is free of all vrittis, distractions and imperfections.

Attempting to describe the almost indescribable, the last shloka says:

Shloka 12

amātraś caturtho'vyavahāryaḥ
prapañcopaśamaḥ sivo'dvaita
evam auṁkāra ātmaiva, saṁviśaty
ātmanā'tmānaṁ ya evaṁ
veda ya evaṁ veda

The fourth is that which has no element, which cannot be spoken of, into which the world is resolved, benign, non-dual. Thus, the syllable Aum is the very Self. He who knows it enters the Self with his Self.

*

The *Katha Upanishad,* among the principal Upanishads, talks of Aum during the interesting dialogue between young Nachiketas and the Lord of Death, Yama.

To Nachiketa's question: 'Tell me which thou sees beyond right and wrong, beyond what is done or not done, beyond past and future?'

Yama says:

Shloka 15, Section 2

> *sarve vedā yat padam āmananti tapāṁsi sarvāṇi ca*
> *yad vadanti,yad icchanto brahmacaryaṁcaranti, tat te*
> *padaṁsaṁgraheṇa bravīmi: aum ity etat*
>
> That word which all the Vedas declare, which all the austerities proclaim, desiring which people live the life of the student of the Truth, that word to thee, I shall tell in brief. That is Aum.

Shloka 16

> *etadd hy evākṣaram brahma, etad hy*
> *evākṣaram parametad hy evākṣaram*
> *jñātvā, yo yad icchati tasya tat*
>
> This syllable is, verily, the everlasting spirit. This syllable, indeed, is the highest end. Knowing this syllable, whatever anyone desires, will be his.

*

The *Prasna Upanishad* refers to Aum in the dialogue between Satyakama and the sage, Pippalada,

Shloka 1

Satha hainam śaibyas satya-kāmah papraccha, sa yo ha vai tad, bhagavan,
manuśyeśu prayaṇamtam aumkāram abhidhyayita,
katamam vā vas a tena lokam jayatīti

Venerable Sir, what world does he, who among men, meditates on Aum until the end of his life, win by that?

Sage Pippalada answers:

Shloka 2

tasmai sa havāca, etad vai, satya-kāma, param
cāparam ca brahma yad aumārah, tasmād vidvān
etenaivāyatanenaikataram anveti

To him, he said: That which is the sound Aum, O Satyakama, is verily the higher and lower Brahman. Therefore, with this support alone, does the wise man reach the one or the other.

*

Many more references to the Pranava are found in the early as well as later texts, but the examples quoted here are important as they show that the teachings on Aum are ancient and also that Patanjali, the author of *The Yoga Sutras* is aware of it. In spite of his predominantly Sankhyan leanings, he is ready to give credence to Upanishadic tradition when required, even though he does not overtly acknowledge his indebtedness.

He comes through as a teacher who is ready to embrace non-Sankhya teachings, provided they contribute to the sole goal of yoga, which is Kaivalya or liberation.

⁕

A brief discussion on Sutra 28 of the Samadhi Pada of *The Yoga Sutras* is necessary now. The sutra says: 'Repetition of it and realisation of its purpose.'

If we look at Aum as pure sound, capable of overcoming obstacles to the attainment of samadhi or pure, inner consciousness, as mentioned in Sutra 29, the question arises as to how it should be repeated or chanted and whether there are certain techniques to do that.

Although strictly speaking, practical methods are discussed more in the section called Sadhana Pada, it would be worthwhile to discuss the practice of *Pranava Sadhana* or repetition of Aum right now since we are already on the subject.

Here is a technique of chanting Aum as learnt by me, an initiated Kriya Yogi. My teacher belongs to the Nath tradition.

Sit in a comfortable posture, preferably cross-legged, on a rug or folded blanket. Face any direction and close your eyes.

Inhale deeply. Open your mouth slightly when you exhale and along with your exhalation, chant a long drawn 'Auuuuuummm,' as long as your exhalation lasts. Then close your mouth and inhale again deeply through your nose. Repeat this exercise for five to ten minutes.

Then let go of all breath control and simply chant for two minutes or so. Now stop chanting and enjoy the silence with your eyes closed. Reflect on the Upanishadic teachings that Om represents your innermost, blissful Self.

Aum should be chanted after practising asanas and just before *shavasana*. Photographs of a whole set of asanas are given in the appropriate chapter. For those who don't do asanas, anytime is good as long as the stomach is not bloated with food. A light snack is okay, but the best results are achieved on an empty stomach, preferably early in the morning.

Another Aum technique will be discussed in the chapter that deals with pranayama or breathing techniques and dhyana or meditation.

How useful these techniques are and what obstacles will be overcome in moving forward towards the goal, we will look at in the next chapter.

I am tempted to use a cliché, 'The proof of the pudding is in the eating.' And this is what Patanjali says in a way, '*nairantarya abhyasena*'—the results come with ceaseless practice.

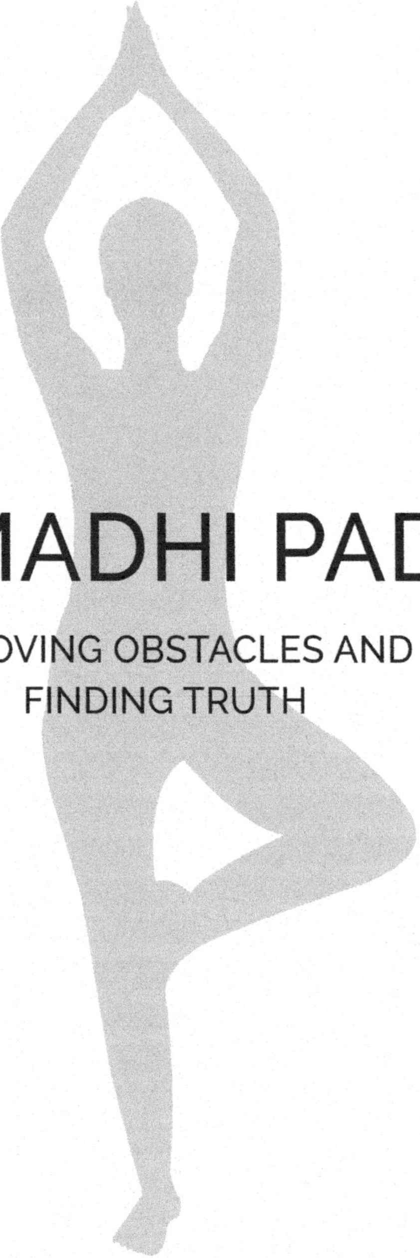

SAMADHI PADA

REMOVING OBSTACLES AND FINDING TRUTH

In continuation from Chapter 4 on the Samadhi Pada, in Sutra 30, which comes next, the obstacles that prevent one from reaching inward consciousness are listed. The practice of techniques like chanting of Aum removes obstacles, one by one, and the mind attains tranquillity. As a result, the inner source of universal power and almost infinite energy is manifested.

Sutra 30

> *Vyadhi-styana-sam'saya-alasya-avirati-bhranti-dharsana-alabdha-bhumika-anavasthiratvam citta-viksepas te'ntterayah*
>
> These obstacles and distractions are sickness, dullness, doubt, carelessness, laziness, some addictions, false views, non-attainment of a spiritual stage and instability.

Sutra 31

> *duhkha-daurmanasyāngam-ejayatva-svāsa-prasvāsā vikṣepa-sahabhuvah*
>
> A dissatisfied, despairing body and unsteady inhalation and exhalation accompany the distractions.

What is to be specially noted is that according to Patanjali, a despairing and dissatisfied person's inhalation and exhalation are unsteady. In order to counteract the dissatisfaction and despair, the practices are listed one after another.

Sutra 32

tat-pratiṣedhārtham eka-tattvābhyāsaï

For the purpose of counteracting them, there is the practice of single-pointedness.

Sutra 33

maitrî-karuṇā-muditopeṣāṇām sukha-duhkha-puṇyāpuṇya-viṣayāñām bhāvanātas citta prasādanam

Purification of the mind can be brought about by cultivation of friendliness, compassion, happiness and equanimity (not only in conditions of pleasure but even in conditions of dissatisfaction) recognition and non-recognition of merit.

The key tenets of the science of Patanjali's yoga are:

1. That the body and mind influence each other mutually. The different postures called asanas (explained in the next chapter) influence the mind by ensuring a healthy body. And more importantly, they regulate the functioning of the endocrine glands that secrete serotonin, dopamine and other neurotransmitters that greatly influence our moods and contribute to the feel-good factor.
2. That the mind when free of distractions and impurities experiences pure, unmodified consciousness called the Purusha, which is supra-blissful and beyond all conditioning.
3. That by consciously cultivating friendliness, compassion and equanimity, the mind becomes tranquil in the midst of all circumstances. Here, friendliness and compassion

are not moral precepts, but active practical methods by which the mind turns tranquil.

One's behaviour in day-to-day life is, therefore, self-monitored and adapted to bring about inner change. This can be defined as outer and inner mindfulness. Yoga rests on the principle that as both are inter-related, they are effective practical techniques to bring about a step-by-step transformation.

Here is a practical example. Stand before a mirror. Observe the expression on your face. Does it look dull, gaunt, sad, angry? Well, force yourself to smile. Think of a funny joke or just bring about an artificial expression of smiling widely or laughing at something, perhaps just at your own comic face. When you are actually happy, the brain activates the facial muscles to bring about a smiling or laughing expression.

It works both ways. When you change your expression deliberately, the message goes to the brain that the facial muscles are in smile mode and the brain links it to the pleasure or happiness centre and lo! happiness is generated and is again transmitted to the facial muscle, and you smile genuinely.

There are other methods to pull one out of miserable, sad states. Note Sutra 31, which explains that a despairing and dissatisfied person's inhalation and exhalation are unsteady.

Sutra 34

pracchardanā-vidhāraṇābhyām vā prāṇasya

One of the methods to restore balance and tranquility is by expulsion and retention of breath.

Pranayama or the coordination of breath will be discussed in detail in the chapter on the eight parts of yoga, Ashtanga.

A simple method which can be discussed here is what is called the *Hamsa* technique.

Sit in a comfortable posture, erect if possible, and closing your eyes, pay attention to your inhalation and exhalation without attempting to control the rhythm in any manner. When you inhale, mentally chant the sound '*ham*' (hum) and when you exhale, chant '*sa*'. After a while, you feel like giving a deep sigh. This is a sign that the meditation is deepening and the mind is slowly but steadily freeing itself of distractions and settling down in peace and tranquillity.

The technique is similar to Vipassana breathing where ham-sa is not chanted, but importance is placed on being aware of the breathing.

Sutra 35

> *viṣayavati vā pravrttir utpannā manasaḥ sthiti-nibandhani*
>
> Or a steady bringing together of the organ called the mind happens in complete involvement with a state.

In other words, by giving complete attention to an activity, which could even be a sense activity, for example, a dance, music, or drama, especially of the classical variety, where emotions and rhythm also come into play, the mind is in an undistracted state and immersed in bliss.

In fact, Indian and Western classical music is designed to immerse the mind in rhythmic sounds and patterns, which take one to heights of spiritual awareness. Great singers, dancers, actors, painters and other creative individuals will vouch for this fact.

Sutra 36

> *visokā vā jyotismati*
>
> Or by meditation on pure light, sorrowlessness is attained.

When one meditates on a light, which is internal, the mind ceases to be agitated and attains tranquillity. In practical meditation, if one knocks the centre between the eyebrows a few times and fixes attention on the centre called *ajna* with the eyes closed, by and by, a blue light appears.

Meditating on that light, one attains tranquillity and enjoys the bliss of total calmness that sets in like a gentle breeze.

In fact, there are schools of meditation that do just that and nothing more.

Sutra 37

> *vītarāga viṣayam vā cittam*
>
> Or the condition of the mind which is free from attachment.

The yogi who sees the futility of being obsessed with something which is not permanent rids himself or herself from mental slavery and becomes free and light-minded.

It is possible to work, love and serve others in this world, without being obsessed, says the karma yogi. As one advances in this way of life, the un-obsessed free mind acquires the capacity to think clearly without prejudice and conserve energy, which is usually lost in obsessive thought and action. One is then able to access a tremendous source of energy within the Self that works for the betterment of both oneself and the world, in a spirit of selfless love and compassion. To put it simply, the yogi lives a beautiful free life without being bogged down by obsessions.

Sutra 38

svapna-nidrā jñānālambanam vā

Or rests on the understanding of dream and deep sleep.

Seeing that dreams when actually dreamt, are as real as the waking state, the yogi learns to live in peace and enjoy the dream experience, knowing fully well that in the waking state, the dream experience vanishes.

Also in deep sleep, the yogi learns to rest and rejuvenate the mind as he or she is already free from attachment and obsession. Such a deep sleep, which is both curative and blissful, rejuvenates all the cells of the body, especially the brain cells.

Sutra 39

yathā-abhimata-dhyānād-vā

Or by the desire to meditate.

Equipped with the different forms of meditation, the yogi longs to be immersed in meditation and enjoy the bliss of an undistracted mind.

Sutra 40

paramāṇu-parama-mahattvānto 'sya vasîkārah

The mastering of meditation can be applied from the smallest to the greatest.

The expert meditator can apply his skills in one-pointedness to understand anything from the smallest to the greatest, from ordinary things to the universal truth.

Sutra 41

kṣīṇa-vṛtter-abhijātasy-eva maṇer-grahītṛ-grahaṇa-grāhyeṣu tatstha-tadañjanatā samāpattiḥ

Such a mind with minimum fluctuations is like a clear, transparent jewel and assumes the colours of the objects near it, and thus unites the (one who) grasps (the thing) grasped and the act of grasping.

The meditator, the object or idea meditated upon and the meditation becomes one and the division vanishes.

Sutras 42 to 51 are a discussion on the different states of mind that result from the practices described in preceding shlokas, culminating in what Sutra 51 calls *nirbija samadhi* or seedless state, where all the potential seeds of distraction and contradiction have been destroyed. And there remains only the Purusha, who is described in Sutra 47 as *adhyathma*, the authentic Self, the unconditional essence of the one being.

In the state known as *savitarka* described in **Sutra 42**, the mind though clear and one-pointed, is still in the realm of words, concepts, purpose, memory and knowledge. **Sutra 43** talks about the next step that is *nirvitarka*. This is the state when the mind is purified of memories from past lives and past experiences in the present life. Everything, internal images and perceived objects in the outside world are seen clearly, free from association with memories that have accrued over many lives.

This leads to a state of *savicara* and then *nirvicara,* which **Sutra 44** describes as subtle states that lead to *sabija samadhi* or samadhi, with the subtle potential of distraction still existing, though not active.

The yogi, persisting in the practice of nirvicara or not allowing the mind to form images based on memories and past experiences, reaches the clarity of adhyatma, the real Self, referred to in **Sutra 47**.

Abiding continuously in that state, true wisdom dawns and as **Sutra 48** states: 'The yogi leads a life of *rtam,* which means naturally occurring truth, righteousness and order, established in the inner Self, fully satisfied and yet leading a meaningful life in this world. This condition, as **Sutra 49** describes, is different from that which comes through inferred knowledge or knowledge heard or studied from other sources. It rests in the direct understanding of the unconditional Self, Purusha, the innermost consciousness which the yogi beholds as the only reality.

Constant absorption in this understanding, which is still considered as a *samskara* or conditioning, however subtle, helps to keep the other *samskaras* or conditionings at bay. It finally falls off when the distinction between the meditator, the meditation and Purusha—the object of meditation—merge and there remains only the Purusha as the absolute entity with no divisiveness.

The last **Sutra 51** of the section called the Samadhi Pada calls this *nirbija* or seedless samadhi.

It would be relevant to take a look at some excerpts from the Upanishads, which discuss what Patanjali deals with in the last few sutras of the Samadhi Pada.

Shloka 3 (*Mundaka Upanishad*, Section 1)

śaunako ha vai mahāśālo aṅgirasaṁ vidhivad
upasannaḥ papraccha, kasmin nu bhagavo vijñāte
sarvam idaṁ vijñātam bhavati iti

Saunaka, the great householder duly approached Sage Angiras and asked, 'Through what being known, venerable sir, does all this become known?' Angiras says:

Shloka 4

tasami sa ho vāca: dve vidye veditanye iti ha sma yad
brahmavido vadanti,
parā caivāparā ca

'Two kinds of knowledge are to be known as indeed the knowers of Brahman declare—the higher as well as the lower.'

Shloka 5

tatrāparā ṛig-vedo yajur-vedaḥ sāma-veda atharva-
vedaḥ śikṣā kalpo vyākaraṇaṁ niruktaṁ chando

jyotiṣam—iti
atha parā yayā tad akṣaram adhigamyate

Of these, the lower is the *Rig Veda*, the *Yajur Veda* and the *Sama Veda*, the *Atharva Veda*, phonetics, ritual, grammar, and etymology, metrics and astrology. And the higher is that by which the undecaying is apprehended.

This is not a call to abandon the Vedas. Sage Angiras declares that the knowledge of the Veda, even if it does not lead to the higher truth, is still considered lower knowledge. By understanding the Vedas with clarity—Upanishad being part of the Vedas—one understands that the accumulation of mere theoretical knowledge is of no use, but may actually act as a barrier to understanding the truth. If this is not grasped, even the Vedas become lower knowledge.

Now, knowledge and memory, which Patanjali says are the last obstructions or coverings that veil the experience of *savikalpa samadhi*, where the Purusha shines forth in blissful solitude, are discussed in another Upanishad. It would be worthwhile looking into it before moving onto the next section of *The Yoga Sutras* called the Sadhana Pada or section on practice. In the *Ishavasya Upanishad*, Shloka 9 makes a rather confusing statement which has often left the scholarly confounded.

Andhaṁ tamaḥ praviśanti ye'vidyāmupāsate
tato bhūya iva te tamo ya u vidyāyāṁ ratāḥ

Into blinding darkness enter those who worship ignorance and those who delight in knowledge enter into still greater darkness as it were.

The first part: 'Into blinding darkness enter those who worship ignorance would be welcome by all those who like to think they are not ignorant but are full of knowledge.' But the second part: 'and those who delight in knowledge enter into still greater darkness', would shock the votaries of knowledge and scholarship, who are according to the *Mundaka Upanishad*, still pursuing lower knowledge.

The first part of the shloka also means that the ignorant go about under the illusion that they are knowledgeable as far as the Ultimate Truth is concerned. This is again referred to in that part of the shloka which discusses higher and lower knowledge.

Among the other reasons is the fact that those who merely possess bookish knowledge often swell with pride, which makes them blind to the understanding of the Ultimate Truth.

One of the last impurities that stick to the mind and which needs to be scrupulously washed away before the mind attains samadhi and rests in the Purusha, as the yoga darshana names the truth, is pride in name and fame. Those who worship knowledge and are puffed up in pride end up worshipping themselves.

The second part of the shloka was explained to me by Sri Maheshwarnath Babaji, my Guru.

Babaji: When you want to understand something, what do you do?

Disciple: I look at it, feel it and read about it and say, 'I now have knowledge about it'.

Babaji: So, you store your knowledge in your memory and when you say you have knowledge about it, it simply means that you can at any time recover the memory of it and say, 'Yes, I know it'.

Disciple: Yes, Babaji.

Babaji: So your knowledge is actually something stored in your memory.

Disciple: Yes.

Babaji: So all knowledge is memory. All memory is in the past. The very word, 'memory' means remembrance and remembrance is from the past. So if all knowledge is memory, all knowledge is in the past.

Disciple: Come to think of it, yes.

Babaji: But, truth, my dear boy, cannot be in the past. It is always the present, right now, not something stored in the memory and recalled. The *Ishavasya Upanishad* declares, '*Ishavasyam idam sarvam.*' Note the word '*idam*, here and now'.

If you worship knowledge, my boy, you are experiencing the past and entering blinding darkness. The Truth is now. See it?

Disciple: I see it. Clearly. May I touch your feet?

Babaji: You may.

SADHANA PADA

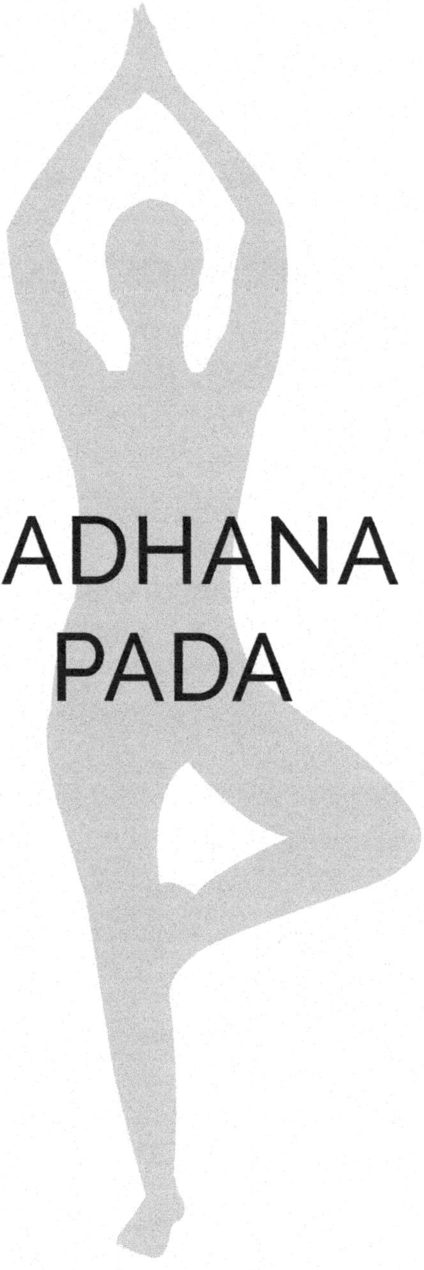

This is the practical section of *The Yoga Sutras*. It deals with the classical ashtanga or eight-limbed yoga, a step-by-step practice manual. However, the previous chapter on the Samadhi Pada, though by and large philosophical, psychological and metaphysical, is by no means strictly theoretical.

A close study would show that the Samadhi Pada also deals with practical exercises like the 'repetition of Aum' and the equalising of the 'inhalation and exhalation', among other practical tips. Nevertheless, it does lay greater emphasis on the psychological and metaphysical understanding of yoga. Without grasping these important aspects, the practical steps would be meaningless, because theory is merely a stepping stone to practice.

Swami Vivekananda's commentary on the yoga sutras, called Raja Yoga, is interesting and relevant to our study.

Commenting on the first sutra of Sadhana Pada, he says 'Those samadhis with which we ended our last chapter are very difficult to attain, so we must take these up slowly. The first step, the preliminary step, is called Kriya Yoga. Literally, this means work, working towards yoga.'

With this introduction, we'll move on to the first sutra of part II.

Sutra 1

> *tapaḥ-svādhyāya-iśvara-praṇidhānāni kriyā yogah*
>
> Austerity, self-study, and dedication to Ishwara are Kriya Yoga.

The word *tapa* is interesting. It literally means 'make hot' or 'produce creative heat'. The synonyms are 'austerity' and 'self-discipline'.

It is also understood that the control of our urge to indulge in sex—*brahmacharya*—builds up inner heat. I can vouch for this. Milarepa, the Tibetan yogi is said to have sat amidst the snows of the Himalayas with just a cotton loincloth, and generated heat enough to melt the snow by the practise of *Tummo*, a certain yogic exercise. My personal teacher, Sri Maheshwarnath Babaji was an expert in this practice and walked barefoot even on the Gangotri glacier.

Swadhyaya is the self-study of those texts that provide an insight into the practices that take one to the Superconscious state. This state is not to be confused with texts that are still in the realm of theoretically establishing the concept of superconscious experience that leads to Kaivalya or freedom.

The yogi at this stage of his journey is understood to have left all arguments behind and would have advanced to the core of that practice that leads to immediate freedom and peace.

The Bhagavad Gita says, '*Upanishadatsu Brahma vidyayaam yoga shastrae*', acknowledging that the Truth—Brahma Vidya—understood by studying the Upanishads needs yoga shastra to be realised and experienced by the student.

Ishwara Pranidhanani—dedication to Ishwara should be understood with reference to the first chapter, where an elaborate discussion on the yogic concept of Ishwara has already been taken up.

Suffice it to state that in Patanjali's Darshana, Ishwara is nowhere associated with a creator God or a controller God and represents the sum-total of all knowledge that has been in existence from time immemorial, and therefore, is the primordial teacher of all spiritual understanding.

The closest one can get to in attempting to define Patanjali's Ishwara is the concept of Purusha, especially the primordial Purusha in Sankhya, which is an aetheistic philosophy and from which the Yoga Darshana has borrowed most of its terms and concepts.

When the yogi reaches the culmination of the yogic process and attains *nirvikalpa samadhi,* then the pure consciousness called Purusha alone shines forth.

It is from this concept that dedication to Ishwara has also been interpreted as a dedicated yogi who has, by realisation, ascended to the status of Ishwara.

But this concept is often misinterpreted and exploited by charlatans who demand abject surrender from their followers and make them utterly dependent on them.

The term *kriyā yogah* here, does not refer to any particular school of yoga, but signifies the need to work (kriya) in one's yogic practices.

Sutra 2

> *Samādhi-bhāvana-arthaḥ kleśa tanū-karaṇa-arthaś-ca samadhi*
>
> The purpose of the practice is to cultivate samadhi and weakening of afflictions.

At this point, it is relevant to take note of the fact that till Sutra 28, the practice popularly called Ashtanga Yoga or the yoga of eight limbs is not mentioned. It is only from Sutra 29 that the practice of Ashtanga Yoga begins. Until then, the teaching centres around understanding the root cause of afflictions, so that they may be dealt with.

Sutra 3

> *Avidyā-asmitā-rāga-dveṣa-abhiniveśaḥ kleśāḥ*
>
> This sutra describes the afflictions that hamper the tranquillity of mind needed to touch the freedom of pure consciousness.

Ignorance, I-am-ness (Ego), attraction, aversion and desire for continuity—the desire to live forever.

Now these need to be studied carefully. The *Brahma Sutras*, Upanishads and the Gita, together called the *Prastana Traya*, offer a great deal in this direction.

The next sutras that follow take up each of these words and explain their meaning.

Sutra 4

> *Avidyā kṣetram-uttareṣām prasupta-tanu-vicchinni-udārāṇām avidya*
>
> Ignorance is the origin or field of all other afflictions, either dormant or inactive, diminished (due to various reasons), overpowered by other causes or fully aroused.

The next sutras attempt to define the word 'ignorance'.

Sutra 5

> *Anityā-aśuci-duḥkha-anātmasu nitya-śuci-sukha-ātma-khyātir-avidyā*
>
> Ignorance is seeing the non-eternal as eternal, the not pure as pure, sorrow producing factors as pleasurable, and the non-self as Self.

As Vedanta declares, the root of the problem is that one considers the unreal, phenomenal world perceived by the sense organs as real as opposed to the real Self, which cannot be recognised by them. The famous 'assertation' often considered a prayer, *Asatoma sadgamaya* 'from the unreal may I ascend to the Real' sums up this idea.

What the Vedantins say is what scientists, particularly neurologists, have begun to say today: That what we perceive and feel as the real world, is merely the image of the world perceived through our sense organs which themselves are inaccurate instruments of perception, and based on which, the mind constructs images and presents to us as 'real'.

Different sets of sense organs or instruments of perception, like the compound eye of the common housefly, can project an entirely different image of the same world. The question that arises is, therefore: what is the reality of even this world we experience and live in, except what the mind projects, which in itself is based on the erroneous data provided by the instruments of perception. To quote the poet Alexander Pope, 'The difference is as great between the optics seeing, as the objects seen.'

The Vedantin, and here the yogi, discards all the relative appearances and sensations and believes only in the Is-ness, which he understands to be pure consciousness, and which the unconditioned mind sees as the one Reality, the Pure witness.

Although Plato doesn't appear totally non-dual as the Vedantin is, this quote from Plato goes a long way in explaining this idea.

'There are two things in the world' said Plato, 'One IS and is never becoming and the other IS-NOT but is ever becoming.'

What does seeing the *impure* as *pure* mean? Here, purity is not a moral precept but the mistaking of the imperfect and relative world as the pure consciousness.

And what is dissatisfaction as pleasure: This is the ordinary mind's tendency to find pleasure in the objects of the senses, only to be eternally dissatisfied, and thereby missing the complete satisfaction of realising that the inner Self is by its inherent nature, total bliss and absolute completeness (*Purna*).

Seeing the non-self as the Self is seeing the relative world as real, and associating one's Self with it when, on the contrary, one's true Self is independent of any adjuncts.

The next shloka further clarifies this:

Sutra 6

dr̥g-darśana-śaktyor-ekā atmāta iva asmitā

The Seer (the conscious Self) and the world seen through the senses when not distinguished, gives rise to the feeling of the wrong I am-ness or ego.

Sutra 7

sukha-anuśayī rāgaḥ

To be attracted is to cling to the pleasurable.

Even when one is often times aware that the pleasure is fleeting—and in the end is the cause for sorrow.

The next sutra looks at the other side.

Sutra 8

duḥkha-anuśayī dveṣaḥ

Aversion is clinging to sorrow.

This means mostly experiencing sorrow. The mind develops the habit of enjoying the familiar pattern and develops aversion to non-sorrow, like the pig that wallows in the muck of its sty dislikes cleanliness. In extreme cases, like that of the voluntary martyr, the mind imagines even the pain of dying to be more pleasurable than the state of living.

Sutra 9

svaras vāhi viduṣo-'pi tathā rūḍho-'bhiniveśaḥ

The desire for continuity which even the wise have is a built-in instinct for survival and pleasure-seeking.

From the coronavirus to the complex developed human being, the desire to not die but to continue and multiply is instinctual. It is linked to the ignorance that physical life is eternal.

This will last until the conscious-awareness is realised to be the real Self and not the body or the outside world, in which it appears almost inextricably enmeshed.

Sutra 10

te pratiprasava-heyāḥ sūkṣmāḥ

These subtle hankerings are to be avoided by tracing back to the origin.

This means that from the multiplicity of the world, one has to trace one's awareness to the unity of the pure conscious Self.

Sutra 11

dhyāna heyāḥ tad-vṛttayaḥ

All these distractions and fluctuations can be avoided through dhyana (meditation).

Sutra 12

kleśa-mūlaḥ karma-aśayo dṛṣṭa-adṛṣṭa-janma-vedanīyaḥ

The whole of existence, seen or unseen, is because the roots of affliction are the residue of karma—action from the past.

Sutra 13

sati mūle tad-vipāko jāty-āyur-bhogāḥ

As long as the root exists, it bears fruit being born in certain conditions, as living and experience generated in life.

Sutra 14

te hlāda paritāpa-phalāḥ puṇya-apuṇya-hetutvāt

These fruits are joyful or painful, depending on the causes: meritorious or demeritorius.

Sutra 15

pariṇāma tāpa saṁskāra duḥkhaiḥ guṇa-vṛtti-virodhācca duḥkham-eva sarvaṁ vivekinaḥ

To the one who can discriminate, the conflicts, the expectation and the remittent sorrow, the opposites of pleasure and pain, the anxiety and the conflict associated with them are all summed up by one word—fluctuations of the mind-stuff, vrittis.

Sutra 16

heyaṁ duḥkham-anāgatam

(Such a one) avoids the dissatisfaction yet to come.

Sutra 17

draṣṭṛ-dṛśyayoḥ saṁyogo heyahetuḥ

All this can be avoided, if one knows that the cause of all these afflictions is the illusion that the Seer and the Seen are one.

Sutra 18

prakāśa-kriyā-sthiti-śīlaṁ bhūtendriya-ātmakaṁ bhoga-apavarga-arthaṁ dṛśyam

The qualities of light, darkness, activity, inertia, the material elements, the senses, and the purpose of experiencing the world and even the longing for liberation are only the vrittis, the ambit of the Seen.

Sutra 19

viśeṣa-aviśeṣa-liṅga-mātra-aliṅgāni guṇa-parvāṇi

What is distinct, the indistinct, the one who feels both, and even the unmanifest *akasa* are divisions of the *gunas*.

The commentaries of Vyasa sum up all the above-mentioned qualities and attributes them as still within the ambit of the Seen.

Sutra 20

draṣṭā dṛśi-mātraḥ śuddho 'pi pratyaya-anupaśyaḥ

Although the Seer only sees and is pure seeing, it appears to the mind to be intentional.

Sutra 21

tad-artha eva dṛśyasya-ātmā

The nature of the Seen is only for the purpose of finding the Seer, the Purusha.

Sutra 22

kṛtā-arthaṁ prati naṣṭaṁ-apy-anaṣṭaṁ tadanya sādhāraṇatvāt

When its purpose is over, the Seen disappears; but doesn't disappear for those whose purpose is not over yet.

Sutra 23

sva-svāmi-śaktyoḥ sva-rūpa uplabdhi-hetuḥ saṁyogaḥ

Samyoga is the non-distinguishing between the Seen and the Seer and seeing, therein the mixing up of the owner (a Seer) and the owned (the seen).

For example, when I say 'my body', I am different from my body, which belongs to me. This is similar to saying, 'my clothes', because I am different from them, but when worn both seem to be one.

Sutra 24

tasya hetur-avidyā

Ignorance is the root cause of confusion.

Sutra 25

tad-abhāvāt-saṁyoga-abhāvo hānaṁ tad-dṛśeḥ kaivalyam

From the absence of ignorance, confusing the Seer with Seen ceases; the escape, the isolation, the aloneness not connected to anything—Kaivalya alone is.

Sutra 26

viveka-khyātir aviplavā hānopāyaḥ

The means of escape is constant discrimination.

Sutra 27

tasya saptadhā prānta-bhūmiḥ prajña

The accomplished yogin is now wise in seven-fold understanding.

According to the commentary of Vyasa, the seven-fold understanding is:

1. That which is to be known is known now.
2. That which is to be avoided is avoided.
3. What has to be attained is attained.
4. The ability to discriminate and discern is.

5. The intellect (buddhi) has realised, finished its purpose, first by providing experience and then liberation.
6. All the fluctuations caused by the gunas have ceased.
7. The Purusha, the Seer abides in splendid aloneness.

Sutra 28

yoga-aṅga-anuṣṭhānād aśuddhi-kṣaye jñāna-dīptir-āviveka-khyāteḥ

By practising the eight limbs of yoga (listed below in the description of Sutra 29), impurity is destroyed, and the light of wisdom leads to discriminative discernment.

Sutra 29

yama–niyama–āsana–prāṇāyāma–pratyāhāra–dhāraṇā–dhyāna–samādhayo–aṣṭāv–aṅgāni

Restraints, observances, posture, control of breath, withdrawing the senses, holding attention, meditation, absorption—the state of awareness. These are the eight limbs.

Sutra 30

ahiṁsā-satya-asteya brahmacarya-aparigrahāḥ yamāḥ

The yamas are non-violence, truthfulness, non-stealing, sexual control and renunciation of non-essentials or non-possession.

Non-violence eventually leads to a stage where one gradually loses the desire to kill or injure. For the yogi who finds joy within, it makes no sense to live a life of lies and deceit and to try to reach the 'Truth'. A lying mind is never a tranquil mind.

Sexual control need not be total celibacy. It means all actions that lead to the Brahman. Basically, it keeps the sense organs, especially the sex organs disciplined, so that all the energy of your life is not spent in sexual pursuit.

Libido has tremendous energy and is a creative force that creates a new human being, which is the result of the consummation of the sexual act.

If this energy can be brought under control to a great extent and sublimated to reach higher and subtler emotions, then the awareness travels from the gross to the subtle and finally to the highest possible, in which the human is transformed into a divine being. This is the whole point of practising the raising of the *kundalini*—the divine, feminine *para shakti* that rests at the base of the spine and is raised by the yogi through the five centres or *chakras,* till it reaches the seventh chakra inside the brain, the *Sahasrara.*[3] The yogi then experiences the thousand-fold spiritual orgasm, wherein all the conditionings are destroyed and there is ultimate solitude and total freedom.

Non-possession or what can also be defined as giving up of non-essentials is interpreted as:

1. Simplifying life so that you don't have possessions to worry about.
2. The gradual understanding that even though we surround ourselves with people and things, nothing really belongs to us. All of us will die and leave them behind. So by

---

[3] A note on Kundalini is there at the end of the book.

developing the attitude of not depending on them, when the time to abandon them arrives, when death is imminent, we won't grieve for them.

We should also understand that everything really belongs to the whole world and we are in charge of only a part of it.

As the *Isavasya Upanishad* says, '*ma gridha kasya sviddhanam* (whose wealth is this anyway?)'

Sutra 31

jāti-deśa-kāla-samaya-anavacchinnāḥ sārva-bhaumā-mahāvratam

On all occasions, under all circumstances of birth, place or time, when practised, then it is termed the great Vow (*maha vrata*).

No matter where and which family one is born into or which place or the period of time one lives in, on all occasions and circumstances when it becomes habitual to practice the above restraints, then one is successfully practising the maha vrata.

Sutra 32

śauca-saṁtoṣa-tapaḥ- svādhyāya-iśwara-praṇidhānāni niyamāḥ

Observances include cleanliness, purity, commitment, austerity, self-study and dedication to Ishwara.

(For the discussion and meaning of Ishwara, refer to Section 1 of Samadhi Pada, Sutra 23, the introduction.)

Sutra 33

vitarka-bādhane pratiprakṣa-bhāvanam

For the bondage occurring from discursive thought, the cultivation of the opposite is laid down.

Sutra 34 onwards is an elaboration of Sutra 33.

Sutra 34

vitarkā hiṁsā ādayaḥ kr̥ta-kārita-anumoditā lobha-krodha-moha-pūrvakā mr̥du-madhya adhimātrā duḥkha-ajñāna-ananta-phalā iti pratiprakṣa-bhāvanam

Violent thoughts that are inimical to tranquillity and cause harm to others, that are done, caused or approved by you; lust, anger or delusion, whether mild, medium or intense, which results in endless dissatisfaction, and spring from ignorance, can be neutralised by deliberate cultivation of opposites as prescribed in the next few sutras.

Sutra 35

ahiṁsā-pratiṣṭhāyaṁ tat-sannidhau vairatyāghaḥ

When in the presence of one established in non-violence, one gives up hostility, gradually.

Sutra 36

satya-pratiṣthāyaṁ kriyā-phala-āśrayatvam

When one is established in truthfulness, then there is a correspondence between action and its results.

Sutra 37

asteya-pratiṣṭhāyāṁ sarvaratn-opasthānam

When established in non-stealing, all that is present or available is like jewels.

This can be explained as follows:

When one ceases to think of stealing other people's possessions, the mind is not ceaselessly scheming to get them. The mind then becomes tranquil and begins to see beauty and satisfaction in the little things one has and in the surroundings. Once established in non-stealing, one becomes friends with the little squirrel that comes every day or the beautiful bird that sits looking out from the branches of the deodhar tree, just outside one's *kutir* in the mountains. No thief can steal the treasures of your heart.

Sutra 38

brahmacarya pratiṣṭhāyāṁ vīrya-lābhaḥ

When steady with the practice of sexual control, vigour is obtained.

This means that if one has a certain amount of control of one's sexual urges and indulgence, the tremendous power, which is otherwise dissipated, is withheld and sublimated into physical vigour and mental creativity. This need not necessarily mean total celibacy as there have been great yogis who were *(grihastas)* married men.

Sutra 39

aparigraha-sthairye janma-kathaṁtā saṁbodhaḥ

When established in non-possession, the knowledge of the how and what of existence is born.

When it is clearly understood, by and by, that nothing belongs to one, since one has to leave it behind at some time and the mind begins to extricate itself from the imaginary world of the images we have created depending on birth, titles, and possessions, it begins to see clearly that pure existence does not depend on the image—the ego. Then, the tranquil mind understands what true existence is, stripped of all the paraphernalia that had hitherto kept it enslaved.

Sutra 40

śaucāt sva-aṅga-jugupsā paraira asaṁsargaḥ

From cleanliness/purity (maintaining the purity of the body), one develops dislike over one's body and also of others and avoids contact with others.

Seeing that the body needs constant cleaning to prevent it from the bad effects of sweat, dirt, excreta, glandular discharges and bad breath, one develops detachment from the body that one loved so much before.

Seeing that others are in the same boat, one tends to detach oneself from others and keep contact to the minimum. Today, this is similar to the steps that are being taken during the spread of this current dangerous viral pandemic.

Sutra 41

sattva-śuddhiḥ-saumanasya-eka-agrya-indriya-jaya-ātma-darśana yogyatvāni ca

And the fitness to have the vision of the Self stems from a mind that is light (resting in Beingness), pure (free of all distractions and therefore), content and cheerful, with one-pointed mastery of the senses (that otherwise keep distracting and creating conflict).

Sutra 42

saṁtoṣād anuttamah sukha lābhaḥ

From contentment, joy is gained.

Sutra 43

kaya-indriya-siddhir-aśuddhi-kṣayāt tapasaḥ

From the practice of austerity (such as exercise, yoga, control of eating habits and sexual discipline), the destruction of impurity takes place and the perfection of the body and senses arises.

Sutra 44

svādhyāyād-iṣṭa-devatā saṁprayogaḥ

From self-study (arises) union with the intended deity.

Through self-study, and I would also say, study of the Self, one reaches union with the sought after deity. *Ishta devata* is generally explained as your favourite deity, but in the yogic context, the word '*ista*' could mean your sought after deity, Ishwara.

Sutra 45

samādhi-siddhir-īśwara-praṇidhānāt

Perfection in samadhi (absorption) comes from dedication one-pointedly to Ishwara.

Sutra 46

sthira-sukham-āsanam

Asana is (sitting) with steadiness and comfort.

In the Upanishadic context, asana is *shad* or to sit down where not only the body but also the mind settles down with no distractions and is at ease.

Since *sthira* comes from the root *stha* (stand), it could mean that steadiness is expected not only when you sit, but also when you stand.

Based on this, a number of postures have been introduced since ancient times, some sitting postures for meditation and some non-sitting ones that aim to bring about proper coordination of blood circulation, breath, muscles, inner energy channels called *nadis* and the chakras which correspond with the plexuses.

Hormonal imbalances, which destabilise the mind, physical ill-health and improper posture, are some of the issues that are dealt with by the practise of the asanas.

For a standard list of asanas, please refer to the *Yoga Pradipika* of Swatmarama. Any asanas not included in this list are of doubtful origin, sometimes perhaps gymnastics which have been added on.

I have listed a few essential asanas in Appendix A with photographs. Attempt only what you can. The sitting asanas are fairly simple. If you need to learn asanas in detail, contact a yoga asana teacher. I would recommend a course at the Kaivalyadhama Yoga Institute and Research Centre in Lonavala or the Yoga Vedanta Forest Academy at the Sivananda Ashram in Rishikesh.

Depending on availability of time, I can also teach asanas since I have been practising them for many years.

Sutra 47

> *prayatna-śaithilya-ananta-samāpatti-bhyām*
>
> From effortless and relaxed posture (which comes from steady and constant practice), the mind experiences endless unity (non-conflicted).

Sutra 48

> *tato dvandva-anabhighātaḥ*
>
> Thus (the mind) is not assailed by pairs of opposites.

Because it is no more conflicted and has learnt to relax, the tranquil mind is not affected by opposites that tend to pull it in two different directions.

Sutra 49

> *tasmin sati śvāsa-praśvāsyor-gati-vicchedaḥ prāṇāyāmaḥ*
>
> In this abiding there is control of breath, breaking away from in breath and out breath.

This is a description of pranayama. Abiding by this means that when one is effortless, relaxed and not assailed by opposing thoughts, the breath becomes calm and almost still and the in-breath and out-breath are imperceptible. This is called *Keval Kumbhak*, *kumbhak* without any effort.

However, the science of pranayama has several breathing techniques that are to be learnt from an authentic teacher who will tell you how to balance the *prana* and *apana* breaths, the *ida* and *pingala* channels and to activate the *sushumna*. I once again recommend the *Yoga Pradipika* for a comprehensive theoretical understanding of pranayama.

The aim is to help you reach a stage where there is no need to inhale or exhale or to hold your breath forcibly. Holding the breath forcefully for an inordinately long time can cause haemorrhage of the lungs.

Sutra 50

> *bāhya-ābhyantara-sthambha vr̥ttiḥ deśa-kāla-sankhyābhiḥ paridr̥ṣṭo dīrgha-sūkṣmaḥ*
>
> The fluctuations—external, internal, suppressed, and according to time, place and the number of times this is done—after practice eventually becomes long and subtle.

With practice of pranayama, the breath becomes long and subtle until it's almost imperceptible.

Sutra 51

bāhya-ābhyantara viṣaya-akṣepī caturthaḥ

The fourth is withdrawal from the external and internal state (of the breath).

While the breath slows down and becomes subtle, the mind withdraws from the activity of physical breathing. It saves the energy normally dissipated in heavy breathing and turns it inward.

Sutra 52

tataḥ kṣīyate prakāśa-āvaraṇam

Then the covering (that covers clarity) is diminished (dissolved).

When the mind's imbalances, distractions and resulting confusion are removed by balancing the prana, all the coverings are removed and the tranquil mind shines forth.

Sutra 53

dhāraṇāsu ca yogyatā manasaḥ

And the mind becomes fit for (one-pointed) attention.

Sutra 54

sva-viṣaya-asaṁprayoge cittasya sva-rūp-ānukāra-iva-indriyāṇāṁ pratyāhāraḥ

Sense withdrawal takes place when the senses in imitation of the mind, which has become dis-attached, rest in their own state of quietness.

Here, *pratyahara* or sense withdrawal from the objects of the world is given a different perspective from what is usually understood. It is not as if the sense organs are first withdrawn from the objects, leading to the mind getting detached. This sutra says that when the mind understands the futility of engaging with sense objects, it rests in its own quietness, and the sense organs imitating this, learn to withdraw spontaneously, on their own.

Sutra 55

tataḥ paramā-vaśyatā indriyāṇām

Then follows complete control of the senses.

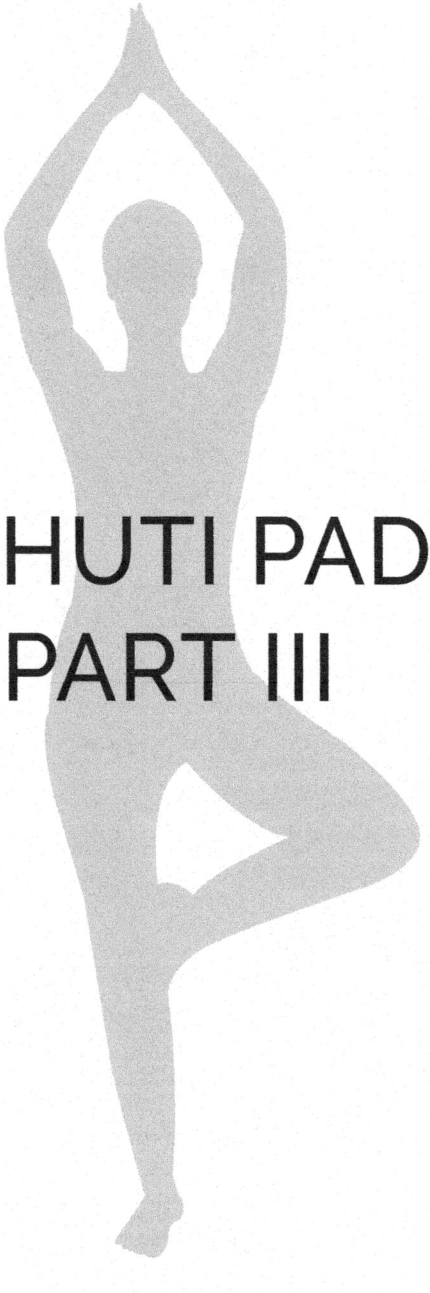

VIBHUTI PADA
PART III

Traditionally, the third pada is about the so-called supernormal powers, but interestingly nowhere in the body of the chapter is the word *vibhuti* used.

These supernatural powers are attained by the accomplished yogi by attention, meditation and samadhi on the object or objective.

Besides discussion on the supernatural, this chapter contains significant information.

Etymologically, the word vibhuti from the pre-fix *vi,* the verb *bhu,* and the suffix *ti* could also mean 'that which is expansive'. It could, therefore, also mean the expansive consciousness.

Now in this context, Sutra 50 is significant—and it is from dispassion towards even these powers, in the very destruction of the seed of desire for powers, that *Kaivalyam* or a state of ultimate enlightenment eventually arises.

Sutra 1

> *deśa-bandhas cittasya dhāraṇā*
>
> Holding the mind to one location is called dharana, one-pointedness.

Concentration, or rather attention is to hold the mind in one place, without letting it get distracted.

Sutra 2

tatra pratyaya - eka - tānatā dhyānam

Extending of this intention is meditation.

Continuing this one-pointed, distraction-less attention for some time is called *dhyanam*, loosely translated as meditation.

Sutra 3

tad eva-artha-mātra-nirbhāsaṁ svarūpa-śūnyam-iva-samādhiḥ

The meaning alone shines, empty of form and that is verily, samadhi.

This can be interpreted in two ways.

1. When the one-pointed attention stretches into meditation, and is reached after a certain depth, the meditator is not aware of individual existence and only meditation remains, empty of even the object that is meditated upon.
2. Through meditation, one becomes aware that all objects and even states of mind are there only for realising the inner Self called the Purusha. When this awareness arises, it's called samadhi.

Sutra 4

trayam-ekatra saṁyamaḥ

The three states in unity—attention, meditation and samadhi—are called *samyama*.

Sutra 5

taj jayāt prajñā lokaḥ

With the mastery of that, wisdom shines forth in its entirety.

Sutra 6

tasya bhūmiṣu viniyogaḥ

This is applied in stages.

Which means, dharana, dhyana and samadhi should be applied step-by-step.

Sutra 7

trayam-antar-angaṁ pūrvebhyaḥ

These three, the inner limbs, are distinct from the ones mentioned before.

Sutra 8

tad api bahir-aṅgaṁ nirbījasya

These three are the outer limbs of nirbija, the seedless samadhi.

Sutra 9

vyutthāna-nirodha-saṁskārayor abhibhava-prādurbhāvau nirodha-kṣaṇa cittā-anvayo nirodha-pariṇāmaḥ

When emergence or extroversion is overpowered by the quality of restraint, there occurs a moment of introversion. This is the result of restrain.

Sutra 10

tasya praśānta vāhitā saṁskārat

The mind then discovers the quality of the mind when there is a calm flow.

Sutra 11

sarvārthatā ekāgrātayoḥ kṣaya-udayau cittasya samādhi-pariṇāmaḥ

When all objectivity is ended and one-pointedness arises, modification (of the mind) leads to samadhi.

Sutra 12

tataḥ punaḥ śānto-uditau tulya-pratyayau cittasya-ekāgratā-pariṇāmaḥ

So again when there is equality of introversion and extroversion between the rising of thoughts and quietness, the result is one-pointedness of the chitta, mind.

This can be interpreted in practical yogic terms as the equalising of the ingoing and outgoing breath, resulting in balancing of the prana in the *Ida nadi* on the left and in the *Pingala nadi* on the right.

Sutra 13

etena bhūta indriyeṣu dharma-lakṣaṇa-avasthā pariṇāmā vyā khyātāḥ

The state of the mind and senses, and the nature of the mind and elements and their engagement with each other are explained and understood.

Sutra 14

śānta-udita-avyapadeśya-dharma-anupātī dharmī

This means that the yogi referred to as the holder of *dharma*, recognises the dharma or characteristics of his mind, whether it is quietened or active or in-between.

Sutra 15

kramāa-anyatvaṁ pariṇāmā-anyateve hetuḥ

The transformation takes place in succession in between these states, causing the difference in states.

Sutra 16

pariṇāma-traya-saṁyamād-atītā-anāgata jñānam

From samyama or a unified view of these three states of arising, resting and in-between, the knowledge of what the past state was and what the future is going to be arises.

With an intimate knowledge of the mind at rest, the mind that is active and the in-between stage, one is able to understand its past influences and what the results will be in the future.

Sutra 17

śabdā-artha-pratyayānām itara-itare ādhyāsāt saṁskaras tat-pravibhāga- saṁyamāt sarva-bhūta–ruta-jñānam

The capacity to distinguish between the meaning of words and their various nuances and meanings comes through samyama.

Through samyama, which is dharana, dhyana and samadhi together, one gets the capacity to understand the meaning behind utterances of all beings. For example, when one praises someone with the intention of flattery, with intentions that are inimical to the person in the future, the yogi clearly sees through the words, however sweet they may sound.

The yogi, through close attention to animals, can even foresee their reactions based on their sounds and gestures. This has been popularly projected as the yogi's capacity to talk the language of animals.

Sutra 18

saṁskāra-sākṣāt karaṇāt pūrva-jāti-jñānam saṁskāra

From perceiving the saṁskaras, one's attitudes and tendencies, one can come to an understanding of previous births.

For example, when a child behaves totally opposite to his parents' behaviour or upbringing, one begins to understand that these are aspects of past births. Prahlada born to Hiranyakashipu is a case in point.

Sutra 19

pratyayasya para-citta-jñānam

From the capacity to see clearly that comes from samyama, one sees other's intentions and there is the knowledge of the other's mind.

Sutra 20

na ca tat sālambanaṁ tasya aviṣayī bhūtatvāt

But this is not without basis, for no condition applies to the physical elements.

What it could mean is that all this is on the subjective level and does not apply to the physical world of elements. Of all of Patanjali's sutras, this is one of the most difficult sutras to translate.

Sutra 21

kāya–rūpa-saṁyamāt, tad-grāhya-śakti-stambhe cakṣuḥ prakāśā asaṁprayoge antardhānam

From samyama—concentration or dharana—comes the capacity to prevent the light rays falling on the form of the body from being reflected in the eye of the beholder and hence, the form is concealed.

This requires a detailed commentary.

The popular interpretation of this sutra is: the yogi, who has learnt how light is reflected off the body, sees the light in the eye of another human being within the yogi's vision. An accomplished yogi can stop the light from being reflected and thus become invisible.

Light rays cannot actually be controlled by the yogi, but the cells on the surface of the body can be made to absorb all the light rays; and in the absence of reflection, the eyes of others cannot perceive the body.

In practical terms, even if one remains still and wears clothes which are different from one's usual dress, and therefore unidentifiable by known people, it's often quite possible to remain invisible. Remaining totally still, though, is not so easy.

Then there is also the fact that in hypnosis, the subject does not see what he or she is told does not exist, even though the object is right in front of the eye. In such a case, the brain doesn't register its existence.

Sutra 22

> *sopa-kramaṁ nirupakramaṁ ca karman tad saṁyamāt aparā-nta-jñānam ariṣṭebhyovā*
>
> From samyama on action or karma set in motion and from observing phenomena that is considered unnatural, there comes the knowledge of approaching death.

This means contemplating on actions, whether performed or not, the yogi gets a fairly clear idea of how far death is from him. Traditional texts also describe the various omens, internal and external, that occur, and by contemplating on this, a yogi knows when death is near.

An example is the rhythm of one's breath.

Sutra 23

maitri adiṣu balāni

By contemplating on friendliness and so on, corresponding powers are attained.

Sutra 24

baleṣu hasti-balā-adīnī

Contemplating on powers similar to the elephant and so on.

Both the mental and physical strength of a human being is not used to its full potential because of the conditioning that the thought creates. It's a kind of self-hypnosis where a person thinks he is weak and cannot do anything beyond a certain point. At times of danger to his own life, the limbic system in the brain takes over and human beings have been known to have performed stupendous tasks for the survival of their own body.

Here, the hint given is that one can improve one's capacity by contemplating on the strength of large animals and by de-hypnotising oneself from the idea that one is weak.

Sutra 25

pravṛtty–āloka–nyāsāt sūkṣmā–vyāvahita–viprakṛṣṭa–jñānam

By the casting of light on activity, there is knowledge of the hidden and the distant.

By clarity obtained through samyama, contemplation, the yogi can see beyond the obvious and learns to read intuitively what the person thinks even though the outward signs are meant to distract. Yogis don't get distracted. So they also learn to see the consequences for the future in the clues offered by the present.

Sutra 26

bhuvana-jñānaṁ sūrye-saṁyamāt

From samyama on the sun and its movements, you can perceive knowledge of the cosmic regions.

Sutra 27

candre tāravyūha-jñānam

From studying the moon, you can determine the ordering of the stars.

Sutra 28

dhruve tadgati-jñānam

By studying the Pole Star, you can determine the knowledge of the movement of the heavenly bodies.

Sutra 29

nābhi-cakre kaya-vyūha-jñānam

By contemplating on the navel chakra in the navel, you can obtain knowledge of the nadis of the body.

Sutra 30

kaṇṭha-kūpe kṣut-pipāsā nivṛttiḥ

By contemplation on the *Vishuddhi Chakra* at the hollow of the throat, you can free yourself of the desire to drink or eat.

Sutra 31

kūrma-nāḍyāṁ sthairyam

By contemplation on the Kurma nadi, a certain internal channel, the mind becomes stable.

Sutra 32

mūrdha-jyotiṣi siddha-darśanam

By contemplation on the brightness in the head, visions of great Siddhas arise.

The centre referred to is the *Sahasrara Chakra* and the Brahmarandhra at the back of the brain centre and the medulla oblangata

Sutra 33

prātibhād-vā sarvam

Having developed intuition, everything subtle can be seen and understood.

Sutra 34

hṛdaye citta-saṁvit

By contemplating on the heart, one can begin understanding the mind.

This refers not to the physical heart but to the *Anahata Chakra* in the centre of the chest behind the sternum. It is actually located in the spine.

Sutra 35

sattva-puruṣāyor atyantā-asaṁkīrṇayoḥ pratyayā-aviśeṣah-bhogaḥ para-arthatvāt-svārtha-saṁyanāt puruṣa-jñānam

Between pure Purusha and perfectly clear *sattva*, there is very little distinction. When this is understood, it is clear that pure sattva is only for the purpose of knowing the Purusha. In samyama or pure sattva, there is knowledge of Purusha.

Sutra 36

tataḥ prātibha-srāvāṇa-vedana-ādarśa-āsvāda-vārtā jāyante

Intuitive hearing, touching, seeing, tasting and smelling of all the sense organs are heightened as a result.

Sutra 37

te samādhav upasargāḥ-vyutthāne siddhayaḥ

In the highest samadhi, there is no desire for even these yogic powers.

Sutra 38

badnha-kāraṇa-śaithilyāt pracāra-saṁvedanāt ca cittasya para-śarīrā-aveśaḥ

With the relaxation caused by the loosening of bondage from the mind, it can enter into another's mind and thereby, into another manifestation.

The mind is capable of entering and understanding other minds and after leaving the body, it can even choose a new embodiment.

Sutra 39

udāna-jayāt jala-paṇka-kaṇṭakā adiṣu-asiṅgah ukrāntiś ca udāna

From mastering the *udāna* or the upward going breath, there is loosening of attachment to the elements of water, mud and thorns and a rising above this.

This is to do with pranayama. By mastering the upward breath that is linked to inhalation, the yogi's mind rises above the distractions of the elements of nature.

Sutra 40

samāna-jayāj-jvalanam

By mastering the movement of *samāna*, there is a glow.

Samana is the breath that balances the upper and the lower breath. With that the body is charged with energy. There is no dissipation. Therefore, the yogi's body and face appear bright and radiant.

Sutra 41

śrotra-ākāśayoḥ saṁbandha-saṁyamāt divyaṁ śrotram

Samyama on the study of the ear and space gives rise to the hearing of divine sounds.

When the mind becomes subtle, it hears sounds, which the ordinary hearing apparatus, that can work only upto a certain frequency of sound, cannot hear.

Sutra 42

kāya-āāśayoḥ saṁbandha-saṁyamāt laghu-tūla-samāpatteh ca ākāśa gamanam

When the mind contemplates on the lightness of cotton, it can move through space like cotton floats when the breeze blows.

Through meditating on the lightness of cotton (wafting in the air), the mind becomes light and is able to move through space.

I am of the opinion that this could mean two things:

1. The mind and the subtle body, by meditating on the lightness of cotton or a feather, becomes light and can move in space.
2. The body also attains a certain lightness and is able to move with ease.

This has nothing to do with levitation, as shown by magicians, which is a combination of mechanical devices and optical illusions.

No human body can get light enough to levitate and all descriptions of the Indian Rope trick are fables or exaggerated accounts of magic tricks and deceptions.[4]

Sutra 43

bahir akalpitā vr̥ttir mahā-videhā tataḥ prakāśa-āvaraṇa-kṣayaḥ

When the outer world is seen without prejudices or preconceived ideas, there is the light of understanding illusions.

Sutra 44

sthūla-svarūpa-sūkṣma-anvaya-arthavattva-saṁyamād bhūta-jayaḥ

From samyama on the gross form and on the significance and connection between the gross and subtle, one wins over the gross.

---

[4] Refer to *How to Levitate and Other Great Secrets of Magic* by John Talbot

The subtle operations that give rise to the gross are grasped, and hence, by mastering the subtle, one learns to control the gross.

Sutra 45

tato-aṇima-ādi-prādurbhāvaḥ kaya-saṁpat tad-dharma-anibhigātaś ca

Therefore, the yogi's increased vision, perfection of the body and nature take place.

Sutra 46

rūpa-lāvaṇya-bala-vajra-saṁhananatvāni kāyasaṁpat

And so perfection of body, with beauty of form, strength and thunderbolt-like solid nature is attained.

Sutra 47

grahaṇa-svarūpa-asmitā-avaya-arthavattva-saṁyamād indriya-jayaḥ

When grasping one's own form and tackling the ego, one finally is able to get mastery over the sense organs.

Sutra 48

tato mano-javitvaṁ vikaraṇa-bhāvaḥ pradhāna-jayaś-ca

Hence, with the swiftness of the mind, when it is finally freed from the conditioning of the senses, the yogi wins the understanding of the originator or source of the manifest.

Sutra 49

sattva-puruṣa-anyatā-khyāti-mātrasya sarva-bhāvā-adhiṣṭhā-tr̥tvaṁ sarva-jñ ātr̥tvaṁ-ca

Once the difference between the *sattvic* and the Purusha is understood, the yogi can control all states of being and is able to understand all of them.

Sutra 50

tad-vairāgyād-api doṣa-bīja-kṣaye kaivalyam

When there is no desire in any kind of power play, when even the subtle seed of wanting sovereignty is destroyed as the yogi realises that it is an impediment to reaching the highest Kaivalyam, then the expanse of blissful solitude is all that he yearns for.

Sutra 51

sthāny-upanimantraṇe saṅga-smaya-akaraṇaṁ punar-aniṣṭa-prasaṅgāt

Being well-established in the right place with quietness of mind, the yogi is able to remain unaffected by thoughts of prestige and attachment having seen the misery that comes out of them.

Sutra 52

kṣaṇa-tat-kramayoḥ saṁyamād viveka-jaṁ jñānam

From samyama on the moment and how it passes, arises knowledge born from discrimination.

By complete attention on when the thought arises and seeing how it rapidly moves on to the past and how another thought instantly arises, which again moves away to the past, the yogi soon finds the gap between the 'thought' that 'is' and the thought that has gone. This gap is the source from which the thought arises. The understanding of this leads him to freedom.

Sutra 53

jāti-lakṣaṇa-deśair anyatā anavacchedāt tulyayoḥ tataḥ pratipattiḥ

The origin of the thought can be traced or known, no matter how different the thoughts are, and hence, can be classified as thoughts pertaining to the past, present or the future.

Sutra 54

tārkaṁ sarva-viṣayaṁ sarvathā viṣayam akramaṁ ca iti vivekajaṁ jñānam

The knowledge born of the discrimination of thought—past and present and the gap between them—is the liberating factor, in all conditions, all times and it is non-successive.

Sutra 55

sattva-puruṣayoḥ śuddh-sāmye kaivalyam iti

When through such understanding, the sattvic mind becomes pure, and there is similarity between it and the purity of the Purusha, there is Kaivalyam (aloneness and total freedom).[5]

---

[5] In Appendix B, please find a simple pranayama exercise.

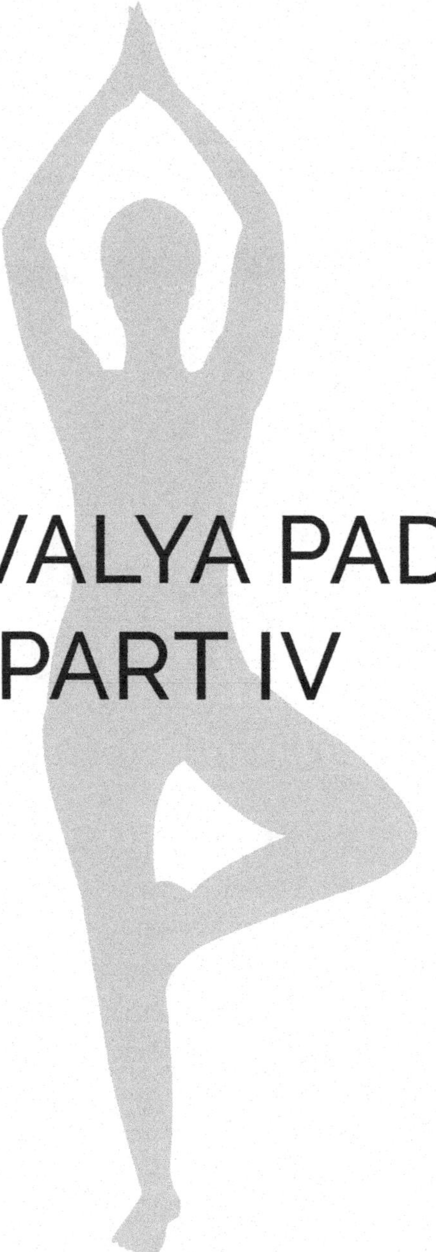

KAIVALYA PADA
PART IV

This chapter is the last of the four sections of Patanjali's *Yoga Sutras*. It describes Kaivalya, the yogi's ultimate goal reached by freeing the mind from distractions forever or eternally. Then only the Purusha exists all 'alone', as the Supreme Consciousness and duality of any kind is banished forever.

But just as in the last section, Patanjali once again deals with vibhuti or 'perfections' described in the previous section before connecting to Kaivalya.

Sutra 1

> *janma-oṣadhi-mantra-tapaḥ-samādhi-jāḥ siddhayaḥ*
>
> Siddis or vibhutis manifest due to birth, drugs, mantra, austerity or samadhi.

What follows is a detailed discussion on the subject.

By Birth

Some human beings possess certain extraordinary capabilities by birth. A classic example of this is a genius like Ramanujan, the Indian mathematician, who came out with advanced mathematical equations with little training in formal mathematics. In the history of so-called spiritual savants, there have been numerous cases of people born with paranormal capabilities. Even some children with congenital defects of the brain have been found to be geniuses in fields like music.

Drugs

It's a fact known from ancient times that certain drugs produce extraordinary states of mind and alter the consciousness temporarily and, in some cases, even permanently.

Alcohol brings about a certain euphoria and many poets and writers swear that it makes them more creative, though weighed against the injury that protracted use of alcohol causes to the mind, one wonders if it's worth it.

Since Vedic times, there has been mention of soma juice, which when imbibed under special circumstances, has caused the user to have visions of other dimensions and divine beings. Except that no one today knows for sure what soma actually is.

Then there are drugs like cannabis, heroin, opium, ketamine and of course L.S.D. which are said to be mind-altering substances, and under certain conditions, expand the mind's horizons, albeit temporarily. Again, considering the after-effects, they are not worth the effort.

A number of so-called sadhus have degenerated into ganja addicts although they might have started taking it as an aid to altering the consciousness to deeper levels.

Mantra

Mantras are certain special acoustic formulas, including the seed sounds, used to invoke deities or special manifestations of the great energy, para shakti, in the six lotuses in the human system.

This brings about the awakening of special capabilities in the yogi. This includes the art of disassociating consciousness from mere body consciousness and expanding its horizons.

Tapah

Tapah, usually translated as penance, is derived from the word tapa or heat. A gross example of it is an animal in heat, when the fire of desire for reproduction rages in his mind. From this is born a new animal.

In the subtler sense, tapah is the one-pointed desire to attain a certain goal in spiritual development, which turns into an ongoing fire that burns away all dross and leaves the essence pure and luminescent.

The penance, performed in the Dwapura, and early yugas like the one Dhruva performed, is unfortunately not possible in this Kali Yuga, where the body cannot survive without food and water.

Samadhi

When the yogi attains samadhi, certain extraordinary capabilities develop following the expansion of the mind, but the aim of samadhi is not the attainment of such perfections but the realisation of Kaivalya or abiding in the non-dual Purusha.

Therefore, the possession of any siddhi is not a criteria to assess the spiritual progress of the yogi, because siddhis are possible through different non-yogic ways.

The corollary to this is that a yogi who attains Kaivalya through the different stages of samadhi need not necessarily possess any of the siddhis.

Sutra 2

jāti-antara-pariṇāmah prakr̥ti-āpūrāt

From the excess of samskaras, of Prakriti, one passes into other births to experience and fulfil desires.

Unfulfilled desires prompt rebirth and appear as samskaras in specific rebirths.

Sutra 3

nimittam aprayojakam prakr̥tīnām varaṇa-bhedas tu tataḥ kṣetrikavat

Like the owner of a field, who diverts water according to his needs, the separation, joining and enclosing of the manifestations is done by the yogi, while the flooding of the water of samskaras from the previous births is not.

Sutra 4

nirmāṇa–cittāniasmitā-mātrāt

The fabricating mind creates images only because of the I-am-ness that it possesses.

Sutra 5

pravṛtti-bhede prayojakam cittam ekam anekeṣām

The pure-sattvic mind that initiates I-am-ness is distinct from the other parts of the mind.

Sutra 6

tatra-dhyāna-jam anāśayam

There, what is born of meditation has no conditioning residue.

Sutra 7

karma-aśukla-akṛṣṇam-yoginas trividham itareṣām

Therefore, the action of a yogi is neither white nor black (no extremes, but is balanced). The action of non-yogis is three-fold, conditioned by the three gunas—*sattva*, *rajas* and *tamas*.

Sutra 8

tatas tad-vipāka-anuguṇānām eva abhivyaktir vāsanānām

Therefore, the manifestation of patterns that habitually occur are caused by fruition of past impressions.

Sutra 9

jāti-deśa-kāla-vyavahitānām apy ānantaryam smṛti-saṁskārayor eka ekarūpatvāt

Since memory is the root of samskaras (past remembrances and their effects on life), they are of one form. Therefore, births, places and times are concealed, but manifest as samskaras.

Sutra 10

tāsām anāditvam ca āśiṣo nityatvāt

There is no beginning of these memories (the beginning cannot be found), due to the eternal continuity of desire.

Sutra 11

hetu–phala–āśraya-ālambanaiḥ saṁgr̥hītatvāt eṣām abhāve tad abhāvaḥ

These samskaras are held together by causes, and the fruits and connection between them cease when there is no more desire. In that state the samskaras also cease.

Sutra 12

atīta-anāgataṁ svarūpato asti adhva–bhedad dharmāṇām

The past and future exist in the mind in their own different forms due to the differences in the paths followed, based on one's dharma and fundamental nature.

Sutra 13

te vyaktha-sūkṣmāḥ guna-ātmānaḥ

These natures manifest with subtle gunas as attributes.

Sutra 14

pariṇāma-ekatvād vastu-tattvam

From the sameness of its evolution (from the same source), there is the 'thatness' of any object.

Sutra 15

vastu–sāmye–citta–bhedāt tayor vibhaktah panthāḥ

Objects though they have sameness, being distinct from the mind, follow separate paths.

Sutra 16

na ca eka–citta–tantram vastu tad-apramāṇakam tadā kim syāt

An object does not depend on one mind for its existence. There is no proof of this: how can it be?

Sutra 17

tad-uparāga–apekṣitvāt cittasya vastu jñāta-ajñātam

An object which is seen by the mind is known or not known because of the anticipation that influences it.

Which means that the mind that has prejudices and anticipations cannot see an object as it is, because the view is coloured by these thoughts.

Here is an example: Because of bad experience in the past with someone, one refuses to see or hear their viewpoint even if it is correct or factual. Anticipation and prejudice colour the world that we see, and so, such a mind can never see the reality of an object.

Sutra 18

sadā jñātās citta–vr̥ttayas tat–prabhoḥ–puruṣasyā–apariṇāmitvāt

The fluctuations of the mind are always known by and are due to the presence of the changeless Seer, the Purusha.

Sutra 19

na tat–svābhāsam-dr̥śyatvāt

The mind with its vrittis is not self-luminous, because it is coloured by the nature of the seen world.

Sutra 20

eka–samaya ca ubhaya-anavadhāraṇam

At any given time, the Purusha and the vrittis cannot be ascertained as being the same, because the Purusha remains distinct from Prakriti.

Sutra 21

Citta–antare dr̥śye buddhi buddher atiprasaṅgaḥ-smr̥ti saṁkaras ca

This implies seeing another higher mind and seeing that the intellect and the subsequent confusion of memory are unwarranted.

This means to try and witness the Self through the so-called higher mind is futile, because the witness, Purusha, cannot be witnessed. It is a witness par-excellence and a mental concoction called the higher mind, which cannot witness it, because there is really no object there to be witnessed.

Sutra 22

Citer apratisaṁkramāyas tad-ākāra-āpattau svabuddhi-saṁvedanam

Due to the non-interference of the so-called higher mind (as discussed in the previous sutra), and therefore, that form or mode being absent, one perceives clearly one's own intellect.

Sutra 23

draṣṭṛ-dṛśya-uparaktam cittam sarva-artham

All meaning is known to the mind, because of the Seer and the Seen.

The experiences of the seen world help to find the distinction between the Seer and the Seen. When the distinction is not seen, there is bondage. When this distinction is understood, the result is liberation.

Sutra 24

tad-asaṁkhyeya-vāsanābhis-citram api para-artham saṁhatya kāritvāt

From actions performed for the purpose of seeking ultimate happiness which is only in the other, innumerable habit patterns are formed (the Purusha though is misunderstood to be for temporary satisfaction of desires).

Sutra 25

viśeṣa-darśina-ātma-bhāva-bhāvanā-vinivṛttiḥ

Seeing the distinction between the modes of action, one for self-satisfaction in the narrow sense and the other for realising the Purusha, one discontinues the cultivation of self-centred action.

Sutra 26

tadā viveka-nimnam Kaivalya-prāgbhāram

Such a mind then, is inclined to discriminate and is not far from kaivalyam, the ultimate freedom.

Sutra 27

tac-chidreṣu pratyaya-antarāṇi saṁskārebhyaḥ

Due to samskaras (past impressions), holes are pierced in the otherwise calm mind by certain intentions (even at this stage).

Sutra 28

hānam eṣām kleśavat uktam

The cessation of even these intentions is like the cessation of afflictions.

Sutra 29

prasaṁkhyāne'pi akusidasya sarvathā viveka-khyāter dharma-meghah samādhi

Indeed, from that reflection, in the one who has discrimination and discernment, only the cloud of *dharma samadhi* remains—the state of tranquillity which is like floating in the cloud of dharma.

Sutra 30

tatah kleśa-karma-nivṛttiḥ

From this proceeds the cessation of all action that takes one away from Kaivalya.

Sutra 31

tadā sarva-āvaraṇa-mala-apetasya jñānasya ānantyāj jñ eyam alpam

Then little needs to be known because of the unending knowledge one has, because all imperfect coverings have been removed.

Sutra 32

tatah kr̥ta-arthānām pariṇāma-krama-samāptir guṇānām

And so, the purpose of gunas (modifications and attributes) is served and done and succession of *pariṇāma* or the results of actions performed is over.

Sutra 33

kṣaṇa-pratiyogi pariṇāma-aparānta-nirgrāhyaḥ-kramah

Succession of thought from the past *kṣaṇa* through the present into the future is terminated by the end of pariṇāma—results of past actions.

Sutra 34

puruṣa-artha-śūnyānām-guṇānām-pratiprasavaḥ kaivalyam svarūpa-pratiṣṭhā vā citi śaktir iti

Thus the return to the origin of the gunas, which are now void since their purpose, that of reaching the Purusha is over. There is Kaivalyam, the 'aloneness' of the Purusha in its original form, steadfast in the power of higher awareness, abiding in the Purusha's, the Seer's original state.

BIBLIOGRAPHY

Taimni, I.K. *The Science of Yoga: The Yoga Sutras of Patanjali.* Theosophical Publishing House.

Woods, James Houghton. *The Yoga-System of Patanjali* with Commentaries: 'Yoga Bhashya' of Ved Vyasa and 'Tattva-Vāicāradi' of Vācaspati Miśra.

Vivekananda, Swami. *Rāja Yoga.* The Ramakrishna Mission.

Feuerstein, Georg. *The Yoga-Sutra of Patanjali: A New Translation.* Dawson & Sons, 1979.

Aranya, Swami Hariharananda. *Yoga Philosophy of Patanjali with Bhasvati.* Calcutta University Press.

Christopher Chapple and Yogi Ananda Viraj. *The Yoga Sutras of Patanjali.* Sri Satguru Publications.

Yoga Sutras of Patanjali in Sanskrit with Commentaries of Vyas and Vācaspati Miśra.

APPENDIX

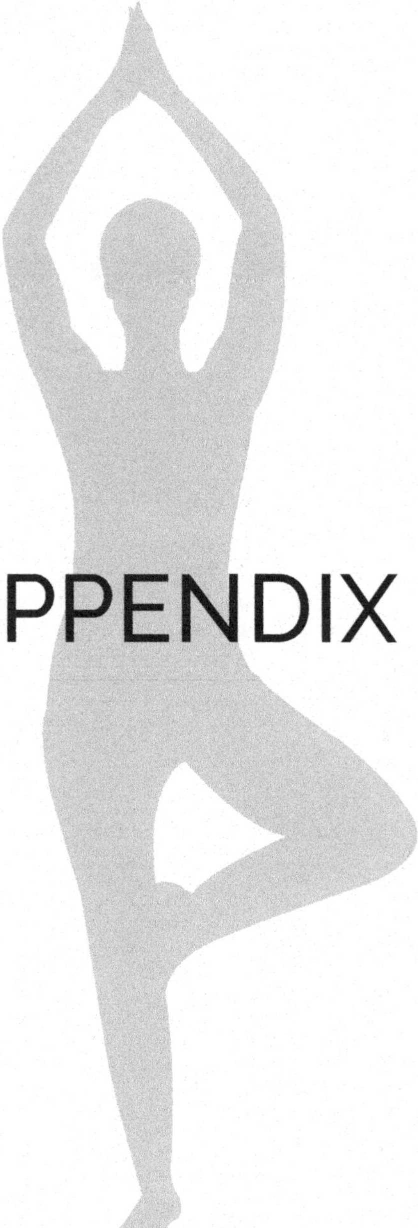

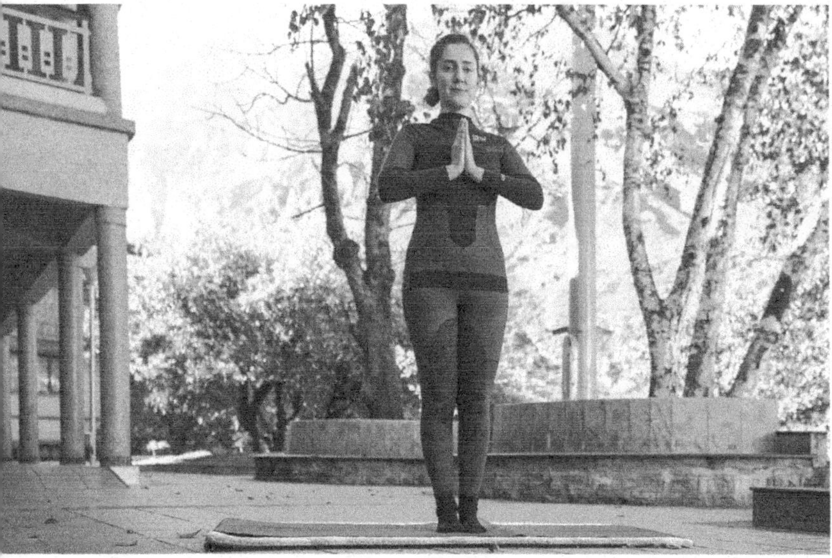

Namaskarasana

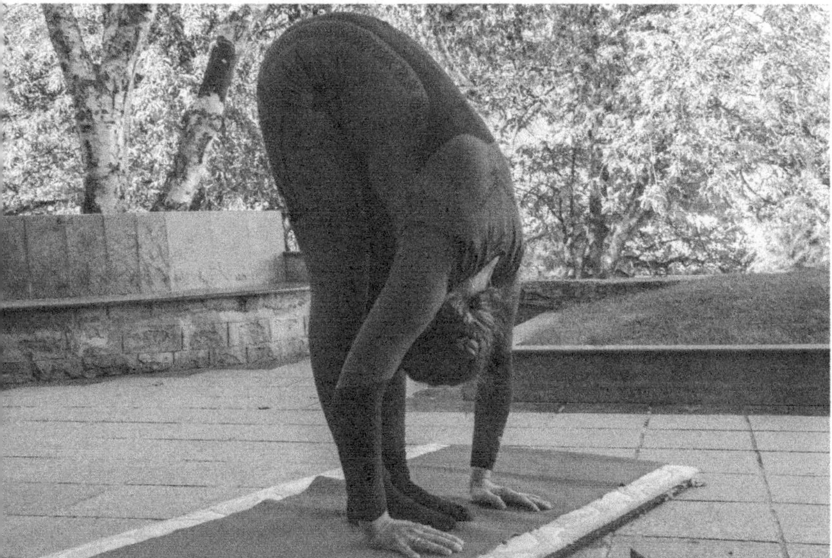

Padahastasana

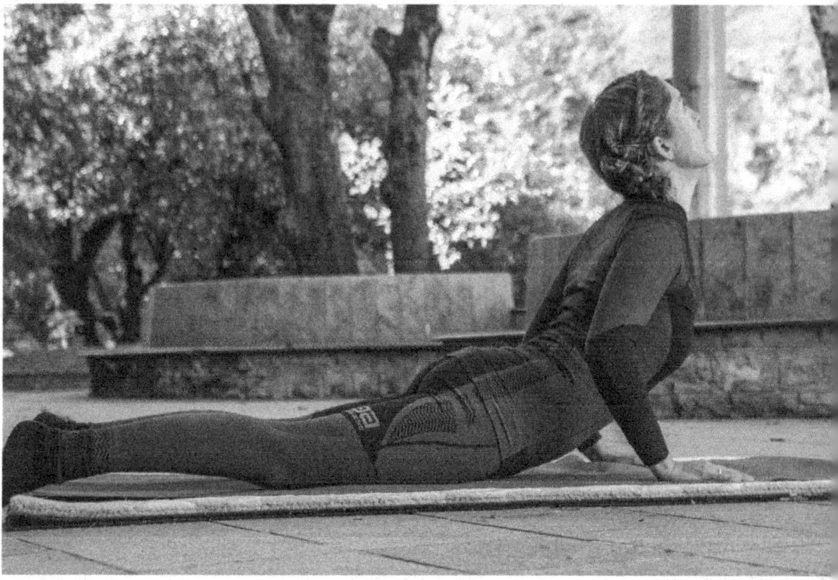

Bhujangasana

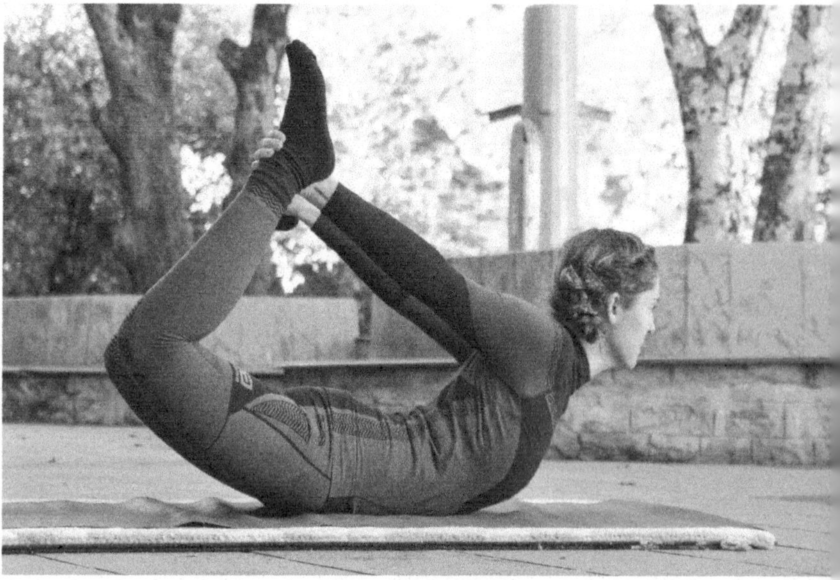

Dhanurasana

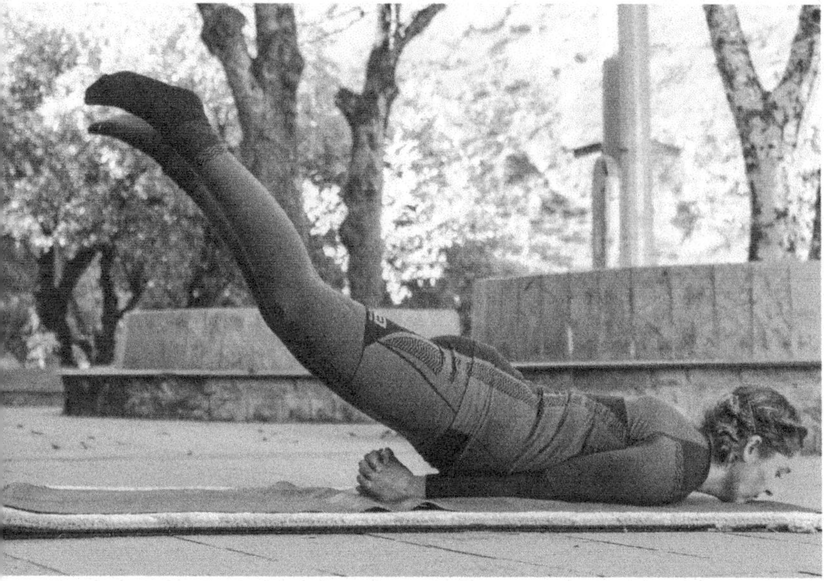

Shalabhasana

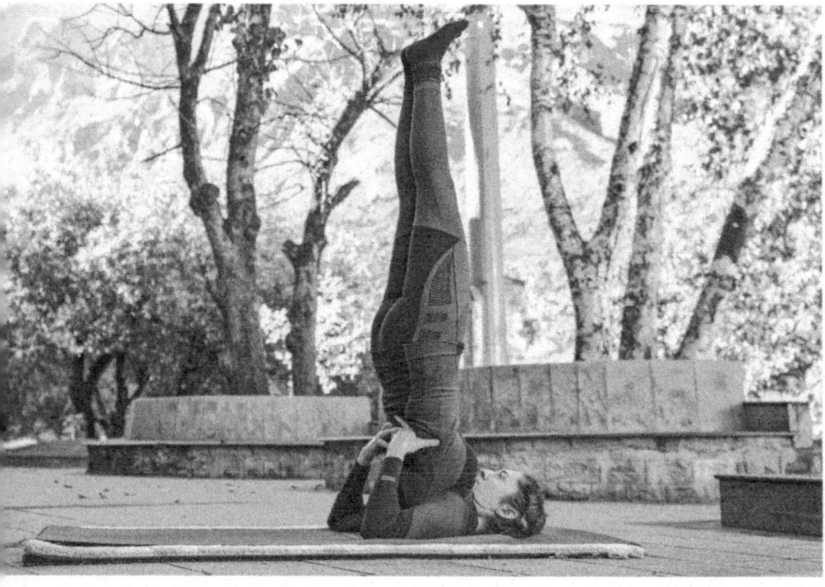

Sarvangasana

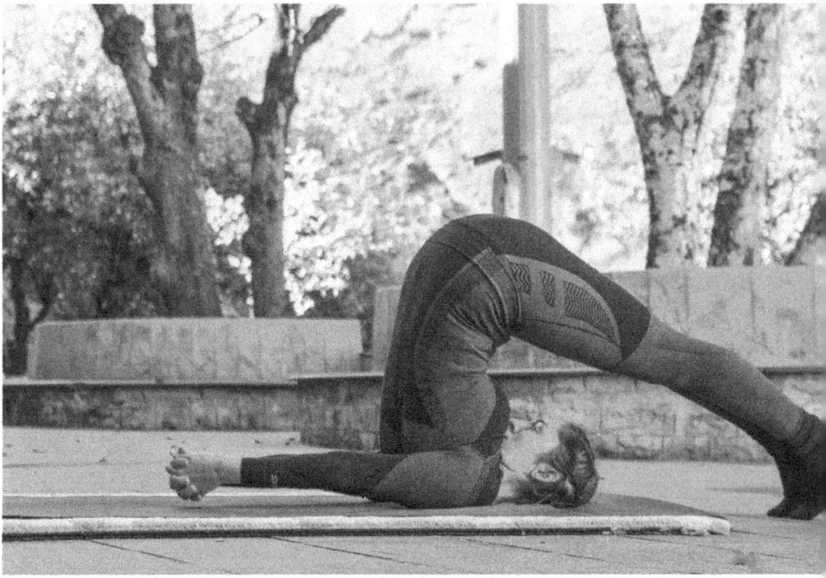

Halasana

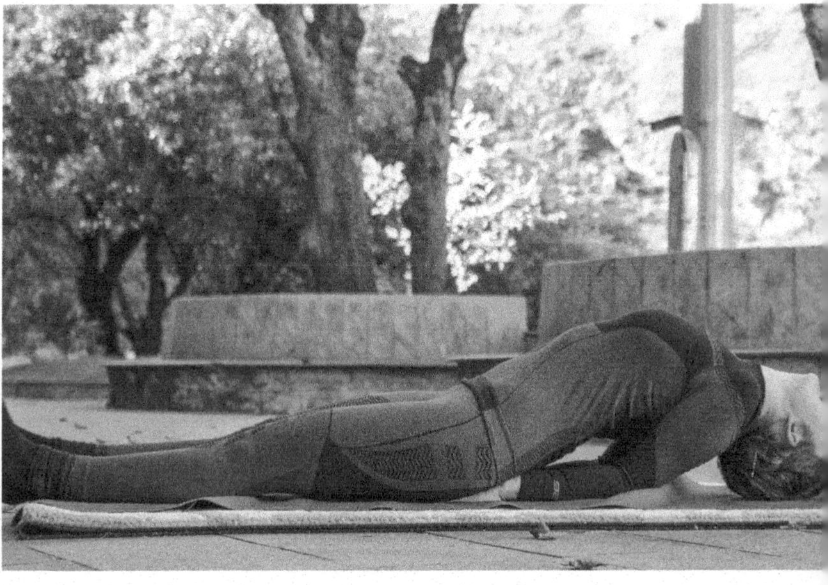

Matsyasana

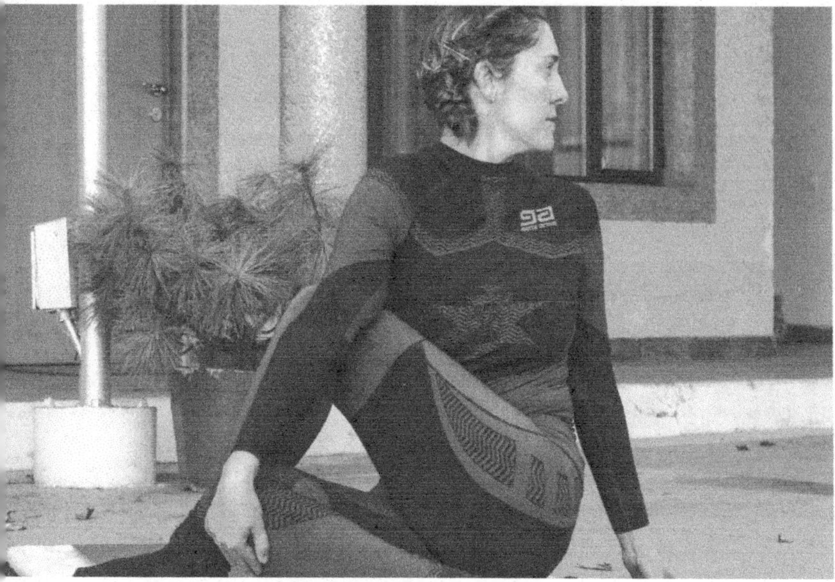

Ardha Matsyendrasana

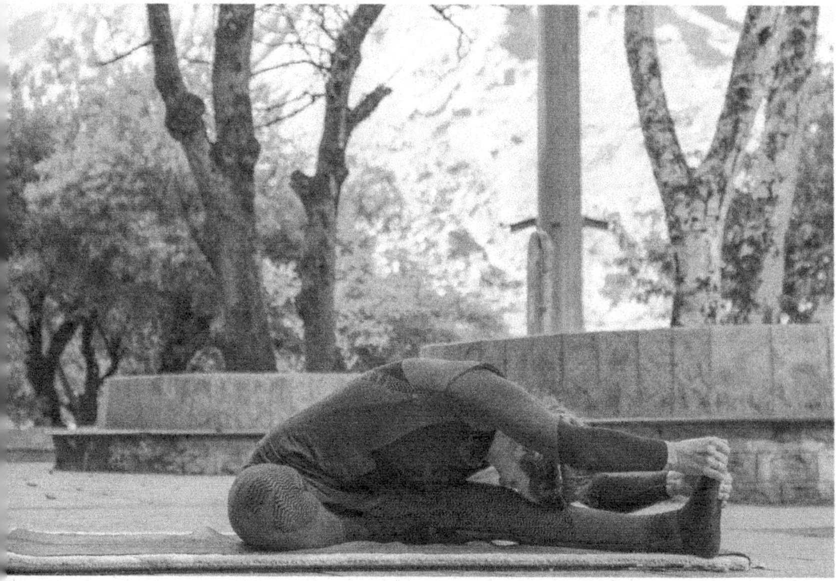

Janushirsasana: left knee

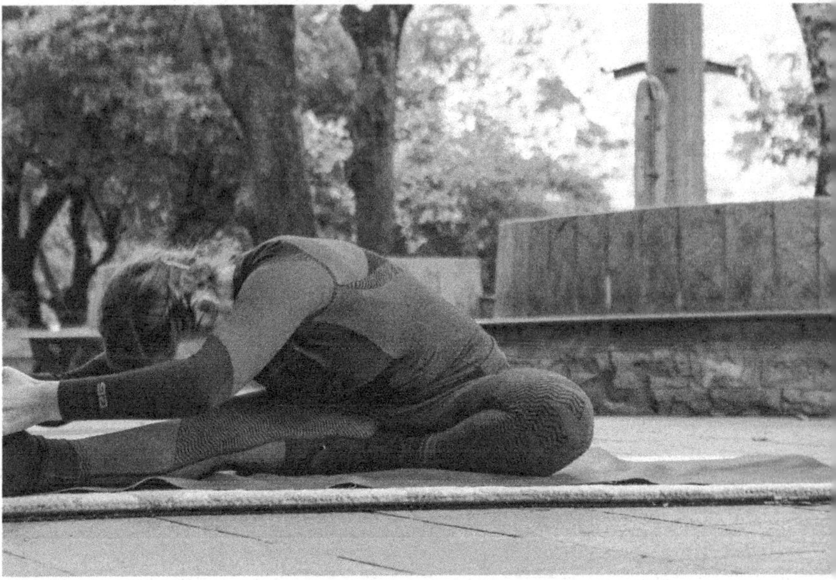

Janushirsasana: right knee

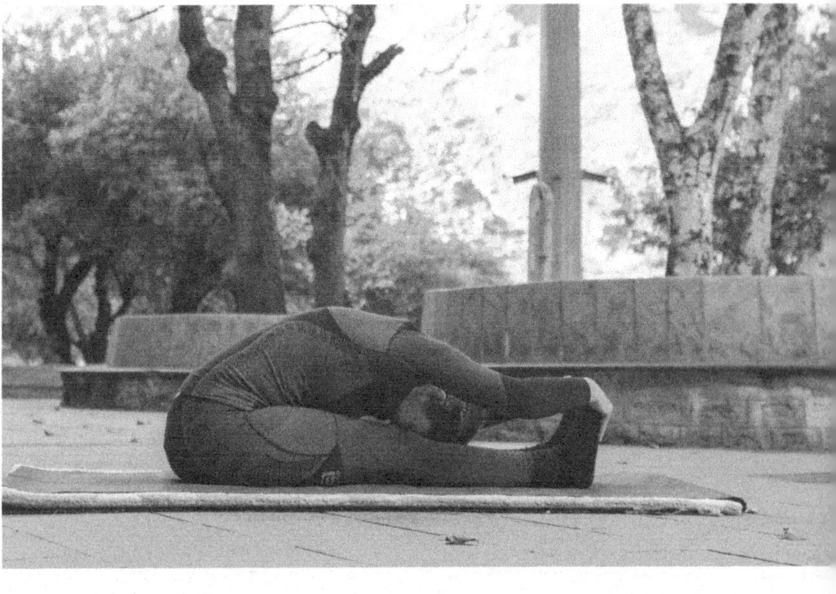

Paschimottanasana

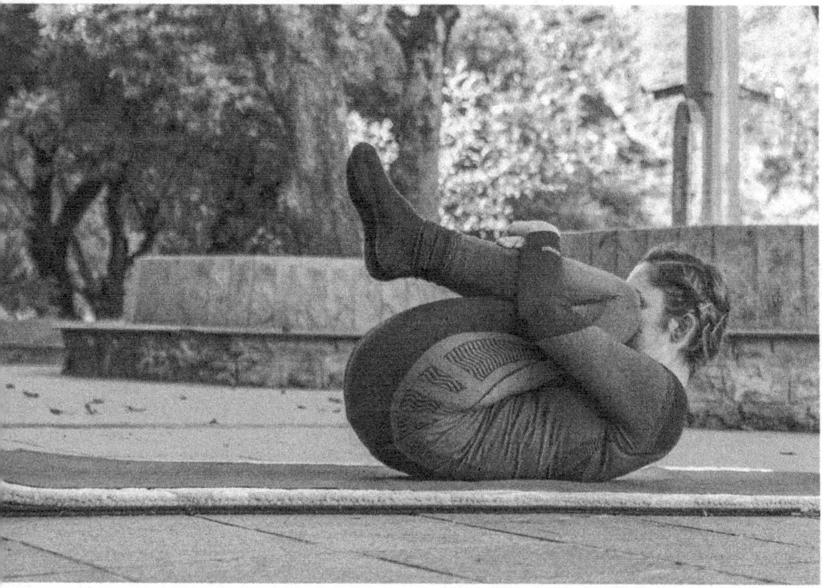

Pavanamuktasana

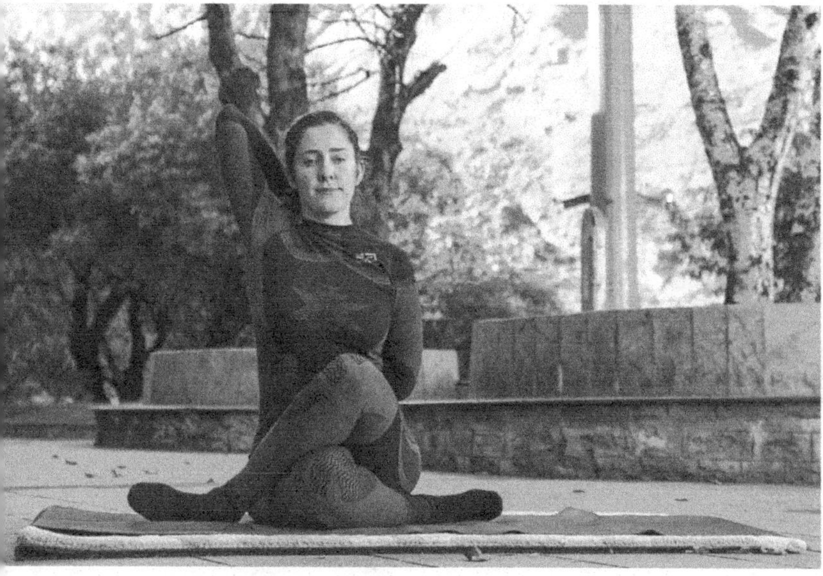

Gomukhasana

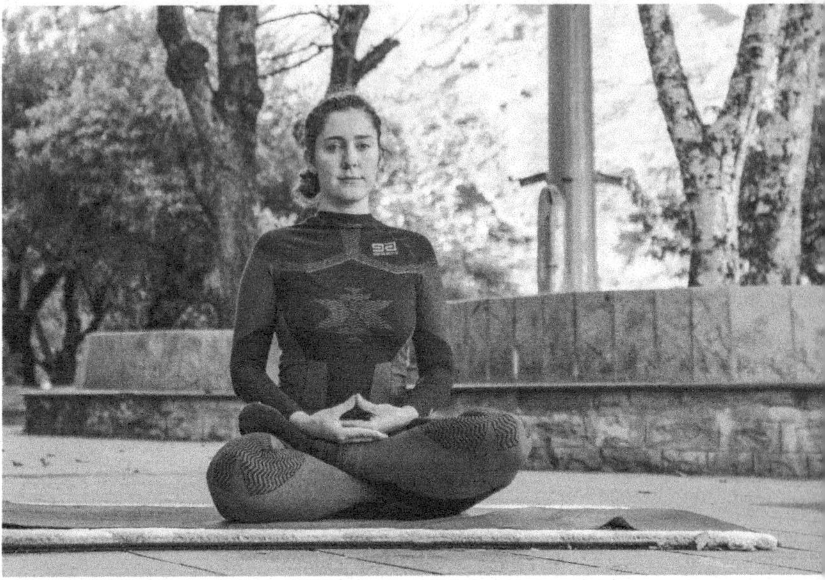

Padmasana

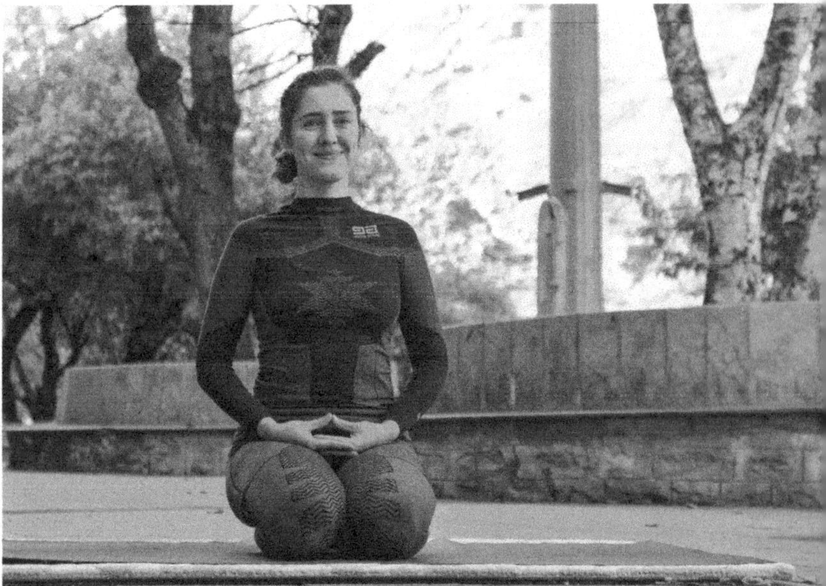

Vajrasana

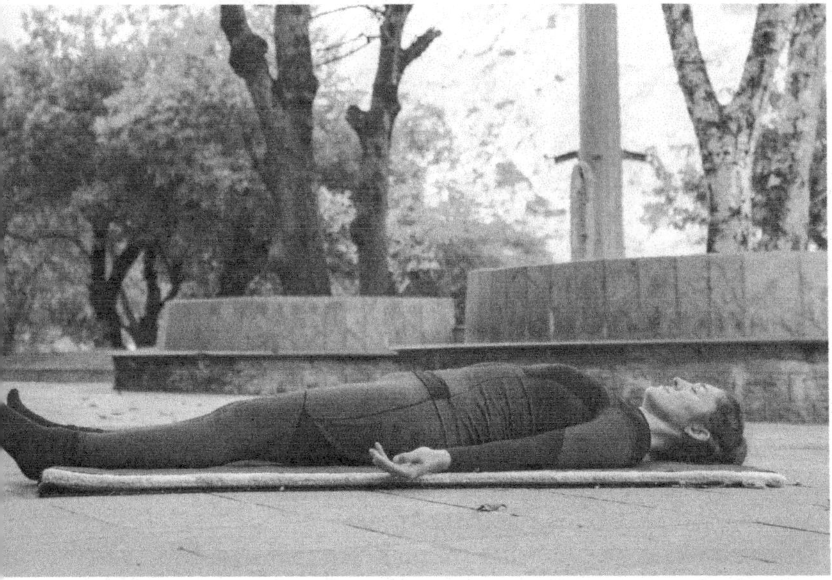

Shavasana

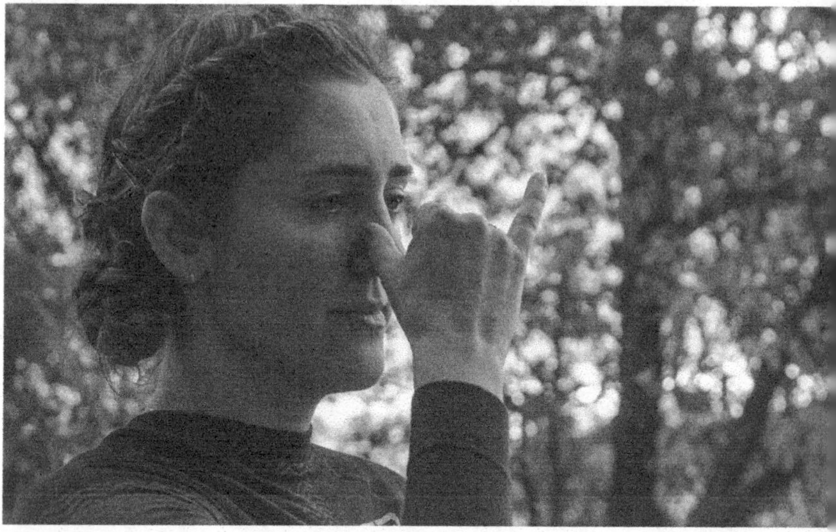

Pranayama: Anulom Vilom, left nostril

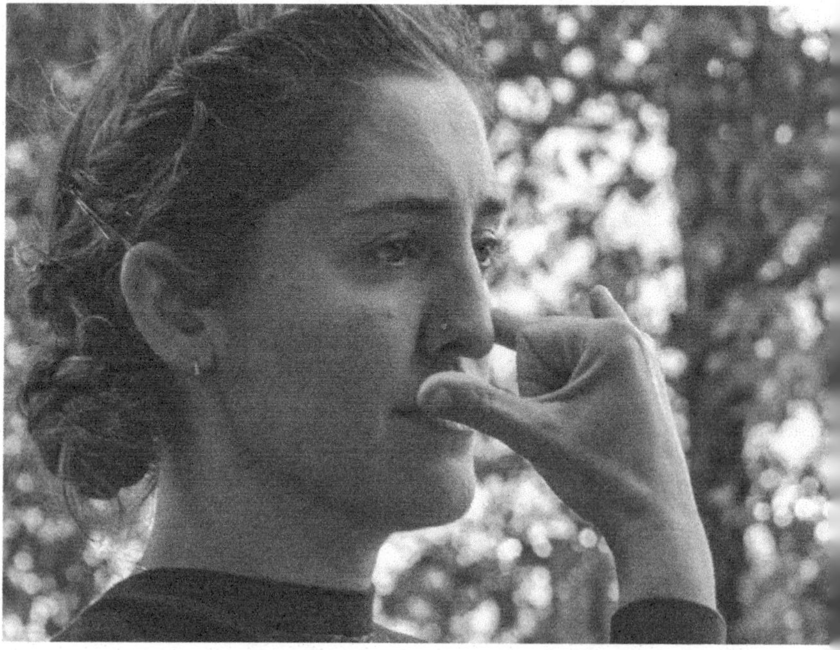

Pranayama: Anulom Vilom, right nostril

Asanas demonstrated by Alina Kaczmarek-Subramanian

NOTE
KUNDALINI

The concept of *Kundalini* isn't mentioned anywhere in the *Yoga Sutras of Patanjali* or in the Sankhya literature. While some of the later Upanishads have mentioned this explicitly, neither the Principal Upanishads nor the various Nath texts like the *Gheranda Samhita, Shiva Samhita* or even the *Hatha Yoga Pradipika* make much of the word *kundalini*. The word kundalini appears in the Yoga Tantras like the *Shat Chakra Nirupana* and other works in Tantra, including the Buddhist Tantras which have predominantly Shakta leanings.

Writers like V.G. Rele in his book—*The Mysterious* Kundalini: *The Physical Basis of the "Kundali (Hatha) Yoga" in Terms of Western Anatomy and Physiology*—have even gone to the extent of identifying the kundalini with the right vagus nerve, which is ridiculous although the vagus nerves have a role in play in the practice of pranayama linked to the psychic pathways. Great Vedantins like Shankara Bhagavatpada didn't mention the kundalini in their major works. Soundarya Lahari which is attributed to Shankara indeed celebrates the ascent of kundalini as the beautiful devi, Tripurasundari. Ramana Maharshi didn't mention the kundalini either.

There are three views regarding the subject:

1. That the theory and practice of kundalini belonged to a secret group of selected individuals of the time and therefore, it wasn't openly and overtly discussed.
2. That for a person on a spiritual exploration of the study, an arousal of the kundalini isn't essential.
3. That even those who don't directly practice the so-called Kundalini Yoga have their kundalini aroused inadvertently with the experiences mentioned in the Yoga Tantras. For example, the experiences of Gopi-Krishna or for that matter, those of J. Krishnamurti; although, he remained silent on the subject when questioned.

I agree with all the three above mentioned points while I don't fully agree with the second point. It would be better to say that the kundalini perhaps is aroused in mysterious and incomprehensible ways during the culmination of the spiritual exploration. Regarding the first point, the reason why the word kundalini has become so cheap and misused is because of the random and freely available—often misrepresented—expositions which have even gone to ridiculous extent of teachers promising to arouse the kundalini in a fixed time for a fee. For those who need a clear understanding of the theory of the kundalini and the description of the chakras or centres through which the kundalini ascends and descends in the human form, there is no better text than the *Shat Chakra*

Nirupana translated by Arthur Avalon as *The Serpent Power: Shat-Chakra-Nirupana and Paduka-Panchaka;* though it must be mentioned that the practical applications should be learnt from a qualified teacher.

To sum up, kundalini, or *Kula Kundalini* as it is mentioned in the Yoga Tantras is the primordial energy, the source of all creation, called *prana shakti* that—after having done its work—rests in the *muladhara* at the end of the spine in all human beings and is intimately linked to the libido. In non-yogis, it is the root cause of sexual arousal, the ecstasy that follows and the biological creation of a new human being. For the yogi, it is the same energy which when controlled and sublimated ascends the centres of consciousness along the spine till it merges in the male component called *shivam* in the thousand-petalled lotus, the crown centre called the Sahasrara Chakra. The teachings for this process can only be learnt from an adept teacher and the results can happen generally only with constant and persistent practice for an extended period of time.

GLOSSARY

1. Darshanas: Six ancient schools of Hindu philosophy. Coming face to face with reality, would be a fair translation of the Sanskrit word, darshana. The six darshanas are Nyaya, Sankhya, Yoga, Vaisheshaka, Mimamsa and Vedanta.
2. Kaivalya: A derivative of the word 'Kevala'—all alone, it means complete freedom from the vagaries of primal objective matter.
3. Yoga: Freeing the mind of all distractions (*yogas chitta vritti nirodha*).
4. Kriya Yoga: A technique, practice or action towards a specific result in the movement towards spiritual fulfilment.
5. Ashtanga Yoga: the eight limbs of yoga as defined by Patanjali namely: yama, niyama, asana, pranayama, pratyahara, dharana, dhyana and samadhi. Patanjali nowhere mentions the term Ashtanga Yoga. In fact, he calls it Kriya Yoga.

6. Vedas: The Vedas are the 'revealed' ancient scriptures.
7. Shanti Mantra: Hymn or prayer for peace.
8. Upanishads: Ancient philosophical texts of India delving into one's true identity.
9. Ishwara: The Supreme Being, a personal God or deity, the Highest Self or spiritual inspiration.
10. Shiva Samhita: An ancient text on yoga which discusses techniques and practices of yoga and theory of 'asanas' or postures as a path towards liberation.
11. Yoga Yagnavalkya: A classical text on yoga which combines ashtanga yoga—the eight limbed practice and Vedanta.
12. Chitta: The mind and the limited consciousness.
13. Vrittis: Movements, activity, distractions.
14. Seer: The subject—Seer—separated from the object, the seen and the act of 'seeing'; a wise person or a sage.
15. Gunas: Attributes present in Prakriti as per Sankhya philosophy which has become the basis for Vedanta, Buddhist and other Eastern philosophies. There are three gunas: tamas (Dark or dense), rajas (Activity based) and sattva (Harmonious, balanced).
16. Abhyasa: Practice.
17. Samskaras: Mental conditioning or impressions formed.
18. Kleśa: Imperfection or affliction.
19. Pravritti: Turning outwards with sense objects directed only to the external world.
20. Nivritti: Turning within or moving inwards.
21. Karma: The principle of cause and effect, action.

ABOUT THE BOOK

Practitioners of the ancient science of yoga have long contended that you don't have to be a Hindu, in the conventional sense, to practise yoga, even though its origins lie in India. Renowned spiritual teacher, author, social reformer, educationist and global speaker Sri M goes a step further in this new and path-breaking book—he proves that, let alone belonging to a particular religion, one doesn't even need to believe in God to be a true yogi. One of the best-known Vedantic scholars of our times, he draws on his deep knowledge of ancient Indian scriptures to prove that the godless are as capable as the God-inspired of reaching the pinnacle of self-realisation and bliss through yoga.

Based on a profound understanding of Patanjali's Yoga Sutras, this is a step-by-step guide to the theory and practice of yoga for those who seek to know it better, and also for the young and the millennial, who may be stepping out for the first time. In lucid prose, with photographs for visual aid, Sri M takes us through the most complex notions of breath, body and posture with admirable brevity and clarity.

If you read one book on the subject of yoga, this is the one to choose.